Basic Arterial Blood Gas Interpretation

Basic Arterial Blood Gas Interpretation

Gary L. Zagelbaum, M.D., F.R.C.P.(Canada)

Assistant Clinical Professor of Medicine,
Pulmonary Diseases,
University of California, Los Angeles,
UCLA School of Medicine, Los Angeles, California

Melvin A. Welch, Jr., B.S., R.C.P., R.R.T.

Program Director,
School of Respiratory Therapy,
Santa Monica College/UCLA Medical Center, Santa Monica, California

Peter R. Doyle, B.S., R.C.P., R.R.T.

Technical Supervisor,
Thoracic Intensive Care Unit,
Respiratory Therapy Department,
UCLA Medical Center, Los Angeles, California

Illustrations by Shelley Hallum

Little, Brown and Company
Boston   Toronto

To my family, Valorie, Nicole, Pearl, Jack, Rochelle, Barbara, Debbie, and Bruce
G. L. Z.

To my wife, Cheryl; daughter, Michelle; and son, Michael for their loving support; and to my students, who provided the inspiration
M. A. W.

To Dad, Mom, Maddy, and Sean
P. R. D.

Contents

Preface

This book is intended to provide basic and practical information that will help in the proper interpretation of arterial blood gas results. It will be particularly helpful to those involved in clinical respiratory care, such as medical students, critical care nursing students, and respiratory therapists, as it provides essential information for clinical management of patients with respiratory and metabolic problems. This is not an all-inclusive textbook on respiratory physiology, but it does include the physiologic and biochemical principles that underlie blood gas interpretation. These principles are presented in concise and comprehensive terms to facilitate the reader's understanding of blood gases.

Each chapter is presented in a particular format. Each page introduces new concepts, defines important terms, or reviews previously presented material. Every page has a key statement that is reinforced by an illustration emphasizing the main concept of that page. Using this approach, we start with basic concepts and gradually build and expand step by step to more complex ones.

Chapter 1 provides information necessary to understand the principles of oxygen and carbon dioxide transport, alveolar ventilation, gas exchange, and acid-base balance. The next chapter details assessment of and factors affecting arterial oxygenation, and what abnormalities may indicate. Chapter 3 describes the importance of the balance between carbon dioxide produced through metabolism and removed through alveolar ventilation, factors affecting that homeostasis, and the significance of imbalance. Chapter 4 details the process of gas exchange and associated abnormalities. Chapter 5 discusses the recognition of acid-base imbalances, related conditions, and disturbances that may result. Respiratory failure and arterial blood gas abnormalities are discussed in the final chapter. Since respiratory failure may be associated with various patterns of arterial blood gas abnormalities, this chapter discusses typical values found in common clinical conditions. There are sample arterial blood gases throughout the chapters and an appendix of problems for the reader to practice arterial blood gas interpretation. Each chapter contains a bibliography for further reading. Terms, definitions, symbols, formulas, and normal values are included in a glossary.

The book's format may tempt the reader to scan rapidly or jump ahead, which may result in missing some key points or subtle details. The reader should try to understand each concept that is illustrated before proceeding to the next page. With time and patience, the reader will master a concise and consistent approach to arterial blood gas interpretation, which should prove invaluable.

G. L. Z.
M. A. W.
P. R. D.

*Basic Arterial
Blood Gas
Interpretation*

1 The Basics

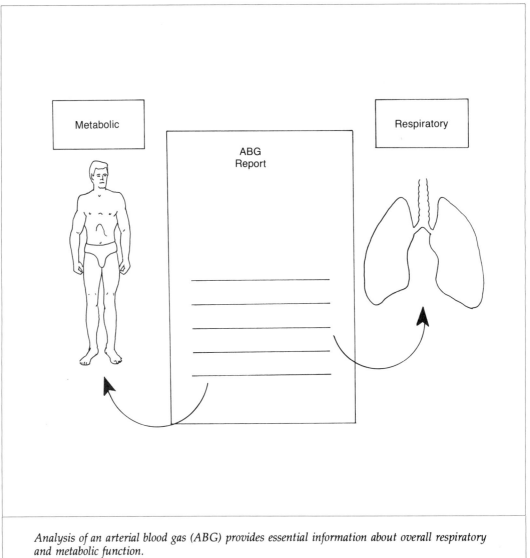

Analysis of an arterial blood gas (ABG) provides essential information about overall respiratory and metabolic function.

ABG analysis gives important information to assist in the clinical management of patients with _____ and _____ problems.

respiratory, metabolic

Note: The most important technical advance in cardiopulmonary supportive medicine in recent years has been the availability of ABG analysis. Modern instrumentation has made these values obtainable within minutes.

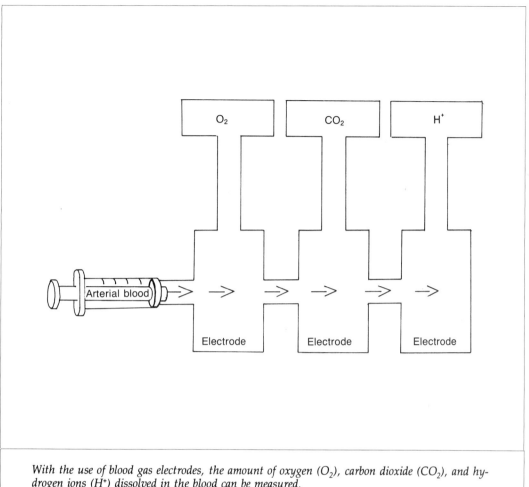

With the use of blood gas electrodes, the amount of oxygen (O_2), carbon dioxide (CO_2), and hydrogen ions (H^+) dissolved in the blood can be measured.

With the use of blood gas _____, we can measure the amount of O_2, CO_2, and H^+ dissolved in blood.

electrodes

Note: The Clark electrode measures O_2 levels in the arterial blood, whereas CO_2 levels are measured by the Severinghaus electrode. The Sanz electrode measures the amount of H^+ in blood.

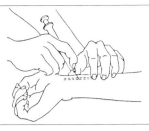

Samples of arterial blood are usually obtained by direct puncture of the radial artery.

The technique for obtaining radial arterial blood samples follows:

1. Make the patient as comfortable as possible and explain the procedure to avoid unnecessary apprehension.
2. With the arm supported (on a table or bed), extend the patient's forearm and wrist as shown above (about 30 degrees). Palpate the radial artery about 1 to 2 inches proximal to the wrist crease. Thoroughly clean an area of skin around the proposed puncture site with an alcohol swab. If difficulty with the puncture is anticipated, anesthetize the skin and soft tissues by injecting 1 to 2 ml of 2 percent lidocaine (Xylocaine) subcutaneously.
3. Fill a 5-ml syringe (preferably glass) fitted with a 20- or 21-gauge needle with 0.5 ml of a 1 : 1000 solution of heparin. Carefully move the plunger of the syringe back and forth to coat the inside of the barrel with heparin. Expel any residual heparin, leaving only the thin coating inside the syringe.
4. While palpating the artery, puncture the skin quickly at a 60-degree angle with the bevel of the needle facing downward and the needle aimed directly at the arterial pulse.
5. Carefully advance the needle until blood appears in the syringe. Immediately stop advancing the needle when this occurs as it indicates you have entered the artery. Allow 2 to 3 ml of blood to enter the syringe spontaneously by pulsatile flow. If you use a plastic syringe, it will be necessary to draw back on the syringe to obtain the sample.
6. Withdraw the needle and apply direct pressure to the artery at the puncture site for a full 5 minutes (or longer if the patient is receiving anticoagulants or has a clotting problem). Hand the sample to an assistant, who should expel any air bubbles and cap the needle with a rubber cork. Recheck the puncture site for bleeding a few minutes after pressure is released.
7. The blood sample should be immediately immersed in ice to prevent the metabolic activity of blood cells from changing blood values. (Once removed from the body, continued consumption of O_2 and production of CO_2 by blood cells can alter blood values.)

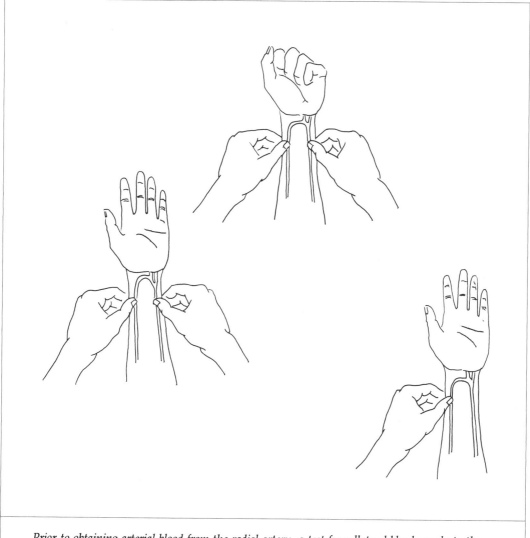

Prior to obtaining arterial blood from the radial artery, a test for collateral blood supply to the hand should be performed.

The _____ artery is preferred for sampling blood because of collateral circulation.

radial

Note: Blood flow to the hand is supplied by the radial and ulnar arteries. When complications occur with the radial artery (e.g., thrombus), blood flow to the hand is supplied by the ulnar artery. The adequacy of this collateral circulation can be assessed by the Allen test. This consists of: (1) applying pressure to both the radial and ulnar arteries; (2) having the patient clench his or her fist firmly, to blanch the hand of its circulation; and (3) releasing pressure from the ulnar artery only. The hand should quickly regain its normal color indicating that capillary blood flow from the ulnar circulation is adequate.

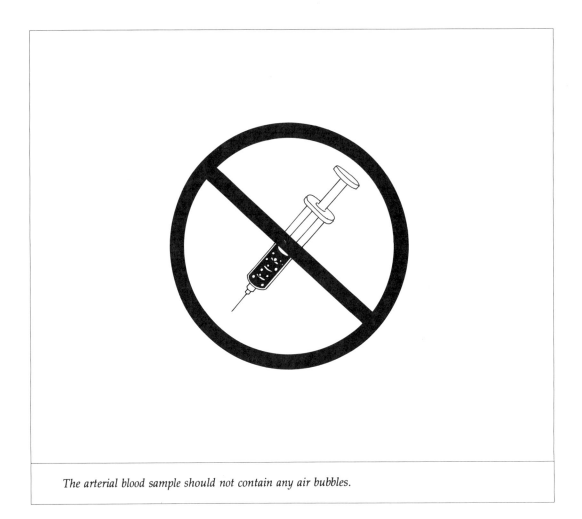

The arterial blood sample should not contain any air bubbles.

Bubbles of air (containing 21% O_2 and no CO_2) in contact with the _____ blood sample will alter levels of O_2 and CO_2.

arterial

The presence of air _____ will lower the CO_2 levels of the blood sample.

bubbles

Note: Exposure of arterial blood to air bubbles could increase or decrease the blood O_2 level. This depends on the amount of O_2 in the blood sample compared with the level of O_2 in the air bubble.

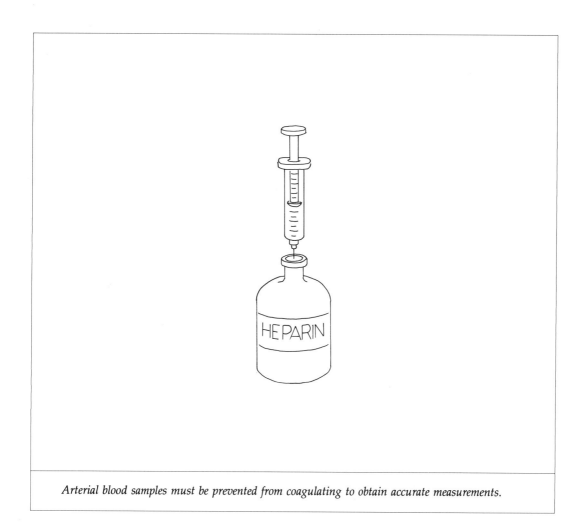

Arterial blood samples must be prevented from coagulating to obtain accurate measurements.

In order for measurements to be accurate, arterial blood samples must be prevented from _____.

coagulating

Note: Heparin is used as the anticoagulant. The concentration of H^+ in heparin is higher than that of blood, while its O_2 and CO_2 values are similar to those of room air. The presence of excess amounts of heparin can alter these blood values through dilutional effects. This is not of practical concern if a large enough sample of blood is obtained (e.g., 2–3 ml) and any excess heparin is ejected prior to sampling, leaving only enough to coat the barrel of the syringe. However, errors could occur if a large syringe (e.g., 12 ml) is used to collect a very small sample of blood (e.g., 1 ml).

The anticoagulant of choice is _____.

heparin

Excessive amounts of heparin can cause _____ in ABG measurements.

errors

7

```
                              ABG Report
Patient's Name _____ Room _____

O₂% _____ Time _____ Technician _____

Patient temperature _____ Physician _____

                          pH = 7.40

                          PaCO₂ = 40 mmHg

                          PaO₂ = 95 mmHg

                          HCO₃⁻ = 24 mEq/L

                          BE = 0

                          SaO₂ = 97.5%




        A typical arterial blood gas report will look like this.
```

Note: The lowercase letter immediately preceding the O_2 and CO_2 symbols indicates the type of blood being sampled. In the above example, the *a* means we are dealing with an arterial blood sample.

☐ *pH* represents a measure of overall acid-base balance and is used to assess the overall H^+ status of the blood.

☐ *PaCO₂* represents the arterial CO_2 level and is used to assess the ventilatory status.

☐ *PaO₂* represents the O_2 tension level in the arterial blood and is used to evaluate the oxygenation status.

☐ *HCO₃⁻* represents bicarbonate, an important buffer in the blood, and is used to evaluate the metabolic aspect of acid-base balance.

☐ *BE* represents the base excess (or deficit) level of the blood and is also used to indicate the metabolic aspect of acid-base balance.

☐ *SaO₂* represents the level of saturation of hemoglobin (Hb) with O_2 and also provides a measure of arterial oxygenation.

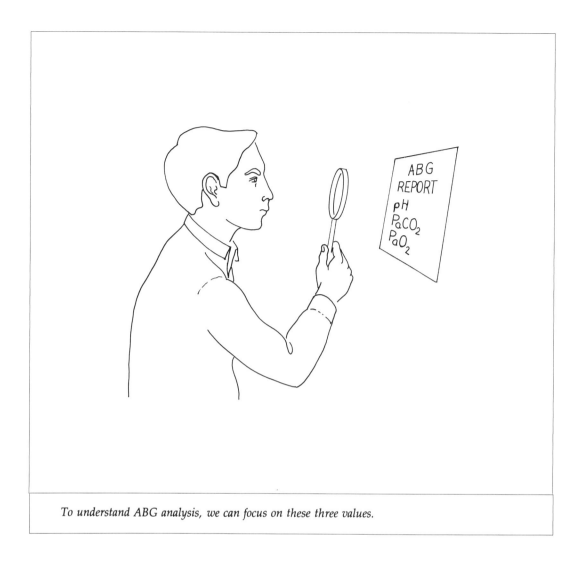

To understand ABG analysis, we can focus on these three values.

The pH is used to assess the overall _____ status of blood.

H^+

$PaCO_2$ is used to assess the _____ status.

ventilatory

PaO_2 is used to evaluate the _____ status.

oxygenation

Note: Although other data on the ABG report can be useful, analysis of these three values provides important information about arterial oxygenation, gas exchange, alveolar ventilation, and acid-base balance.

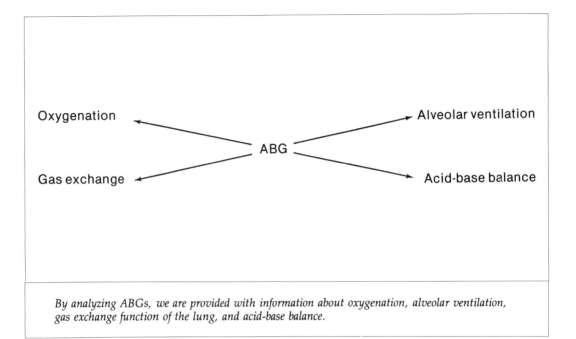

By analyzing ABGs, we are provided with information about oxygenation, alveolar ventilation, gas exchange function of the lung, and acid-base balance.

Note: The term *oxygenation* refers to the process of delivering O_2 to the arterial blood. Alveolar ventilation is the process by which CO_2 is removed from the lungs and O_2 is delivered by the movement of gas in and out of alveoli. *Gas exchange* refers to movement of O_2 from the lungs to the blood and CO_2 from blood to the lungs. These gases also exchange between blood and tissues, and this is referred to as *internal respiration*.

Analysis of the _____ provides a measure of the oxygenation of arterial blood.

The effectiveness of alveolar ventilation can be determined by analysis of the _____.

ABG analysis is also used to determine _____ balance.

PaO$_2$

PaCO$_2$

acid-base

Note: Acid-base balance refers to the net degree of acidity or alkalinity of the blood. This balance depends on the interplay of respiratory and metabolic factors and is reflected in the pH of the arterial blood (see Chap. 5).

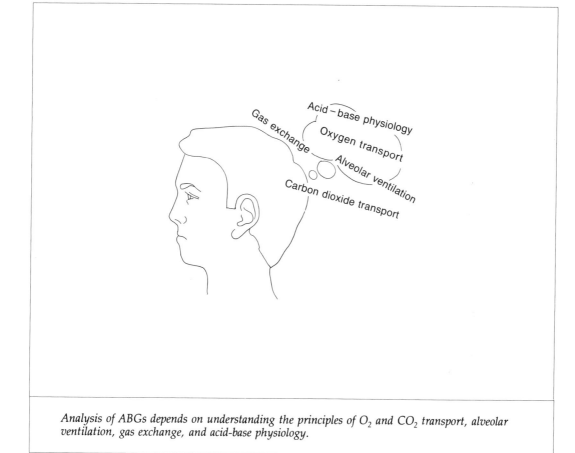

Analysis of ABGs depends on understanding the principles of O_2 and CO_2 transport, alveolar ventilation, gas exchange, and acid-base physiology.

To analyze an ABG, it is important to understand how
_____ and CO_2 gas are transported in the blood.

O_2

Determination of the metabolic and respiratory components of
_____ balance is an important part of ABG analysis.

acid-base

Gas exchange refers to the movement of _____ from
the alveoli into the blood and the movement of _____
out of the blood into the alveoli.

O_2
CO_2

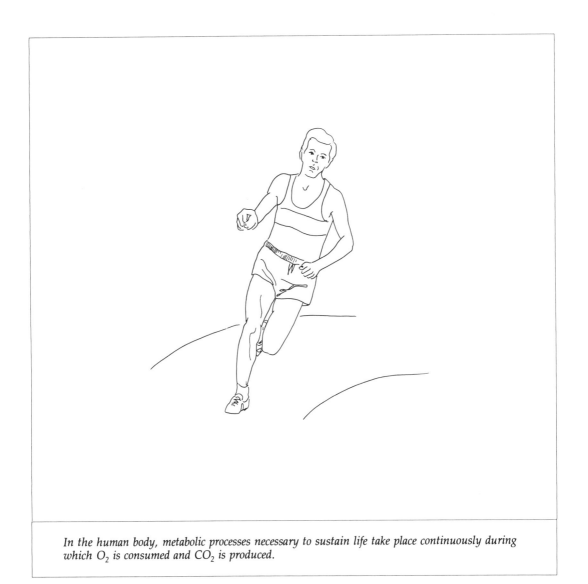

In the human body, metabolic processes necessary to sustain life take place continuously during which O_2 is consumed and CO_2 is produced.

_____ is the gas consumed by cells during metabolism.   *O_2*

A by-product of metabolism is _____ gas.   *CO_2*

Note: Normally, energy is efficiently produced by cells during oxidative (aerobic) metabolism. This process consumes O_2 and produces CO_2. Without O_2, energy production is very inefficient and very little energy can be produced (i.e., anaerobic metabolism). Under these circumstances, a troublesome by-product known as lactic acid is also produced. This acid is harmful to the body's acid-base balance and is much more difficult to eliminate from the body than CO_2.

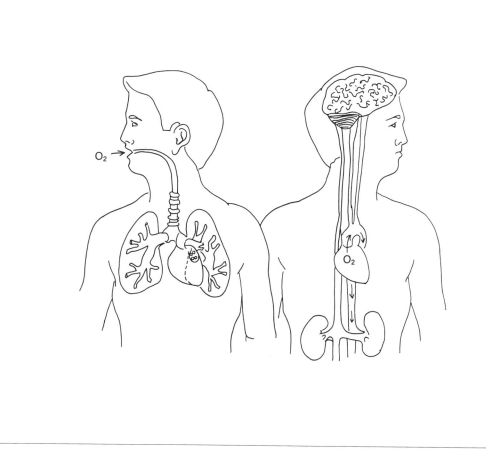

For life-sustaining metabolic processes to occur, O_2 must pass from the atmosphere into the lungs, diffuse into the blood, and be delivered to the tissues by the cardiovascular system.

To reach the tissues, O_2 from the _____ is first inhaled into the lungs.

atmosphere

Once in the lungs, O_2 _____ into the pulmonary capillary blood.

diffuses

Note: This is the process by which venous blood becomes arterialized.

Once arterialized, O_2-enriched blood is delivered to the _____ by the cardiovascular system.

tissues

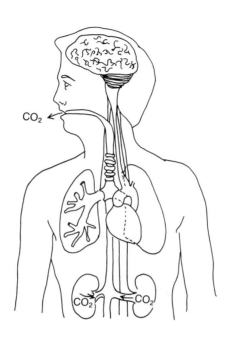

CO₂ produced by metabolism must pass from tissues to the venous blood and then to the lungs where it can be removed by alveolar ventilation.

To maintain equilibrium, CO_2 produced during _____ is removed from the body.

metabolism

The CO_2 produced by cells first passes from the tissues into the _____ blood.

venous

Venous blood then passes through the heart and into the capillaries of the lungs where the CO_2 is eliminated through the process of _____ ventilation.

alveolar

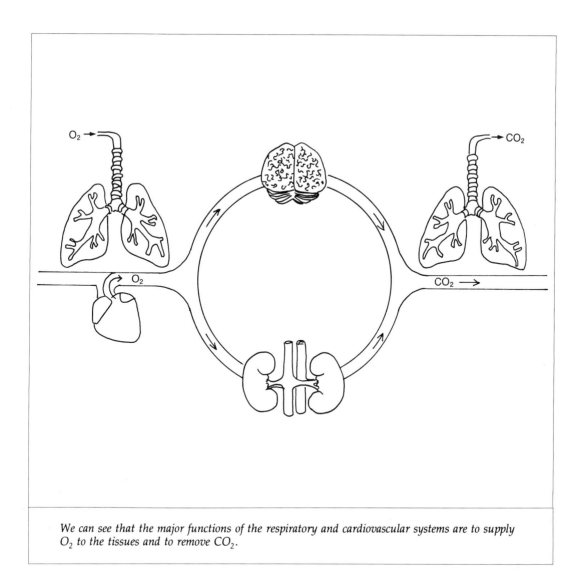

We can see that the major functions of the respiratory and cardiovascular systems are to supply O_2 to the tissues and to remove CO_2.

The respiratory system serves to exchange _____ and _____ between the blood and atmosphere. O_2 CO_2

The _____ system provides the transport mechanism for gases to be carried in blood between the tissues and lungs. *cardiovascular*

By analyzing an ABG, we are provided with information about overall respiratory and _____ functions. *metabolic*

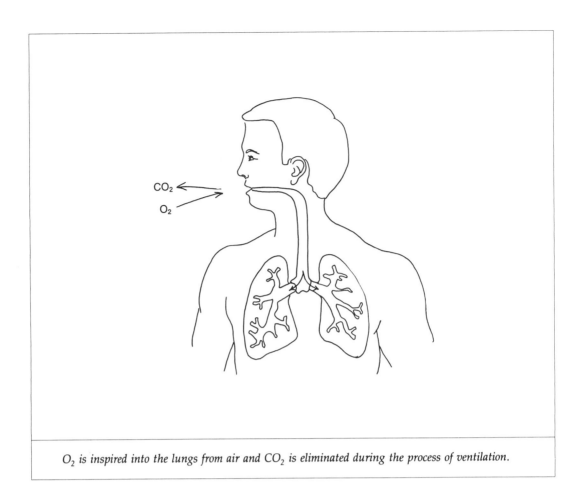

O₂ is inspired into the lungs from air and CO₂ is eliminated during the process of ventilation.

During the process of ventilation, O_2 enters the lungs and
_____ is eliminated.

CO_2

Note: The total amount of air entering the respiratory tract in 1 minute is called the *minute ventilation*. This includes gas that stays in the upper airways and gas that enters the alveoli. The gas that fills the airways leading to the alveoli is referred to as *dead space ventilation* because it does not contribute to the exchange of gases between the air and blood. The gas that actually enters the gas-exchange area of lung (the alveoli) is referred to as the *alveolar ventilation*.

Minute ventilation actually consists of _____ types of ventilation.

two

Both alveolar and _____ ventilation contribute to the minute ventilation.

dead space

The alveolar ventilation is responsible for elimination of

_____ .

CO_2

16

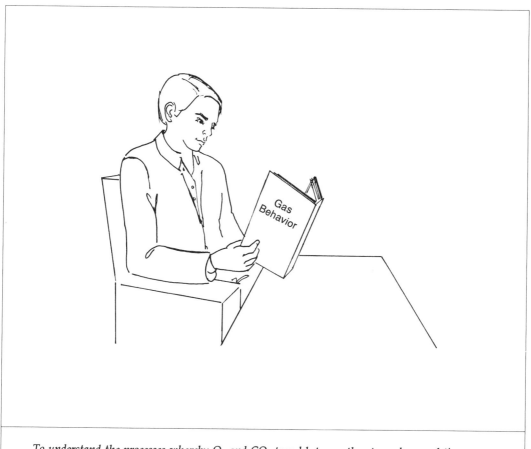

To understand the processes whereby O_2 and CO_2 travel between the atmosphere and tissues, we must first understand the physical behavior of gases.

One of the physical properties of _____ molecules is that they are constantly in rapid and random motion.

gas

Because of this constant _____, gases fill any container they are in.

motion

Note: Gas molecule collisions are perfectly ''elastic'' in that they do not lose any energy or slow down when they collide with surfaces. Have you ever heard of a gas settling to the bottom of a container?

As a result of this constant movement, gas _____ will move from an area of high concentration to an area of lower concentration in a process referred to as *diffusion*.

molecules

Note: Although gas molecules do have mass, they are so small that we describe their behavior as if they did not occupy any space (this is referred to as *ideal gas* behavior).

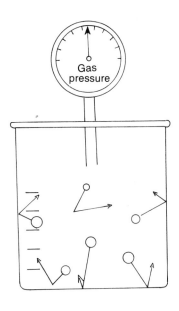

When molecules of gas collide with their container, they exert pressure; the amount of pressure depends on the frequency of collisions.

Pressure is the force exerted by gas molecules _____ with other surfaces.

colliding

Note: In physiology, pressure is often expressed in units of mmHg or torr. The symbol used to represent the pressure of a gas is the letter P. The pressure that any gas exerts when mixed with other gases is called the *partial pressure* of that gas. For example, the partial pressure of O_2 in air is referred to as the PO_2.

As the number of collisions increase, the amount of _____ increases.

pressure

An increase in the number of collisions can result from either an increase in the number of gas _____ or from an increase in the movement of existing molecules.

molecules

Note: An increase in the movement of gas molecules occurs as the temperature of the gas increases.

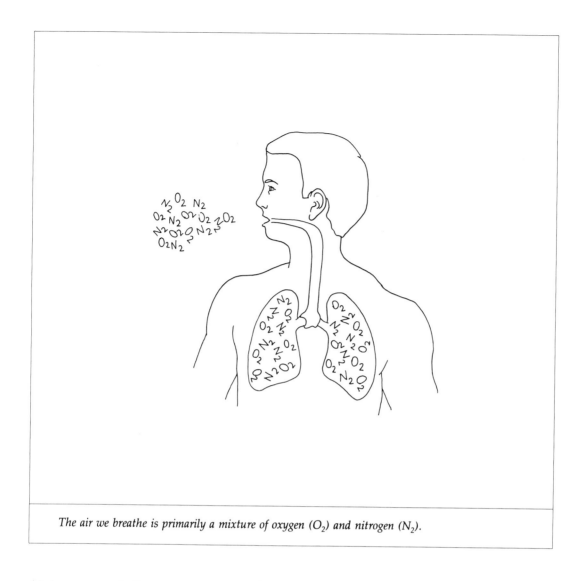

The air we breathe is primarily a mixture of oxygen (O_2) and nitrogen (N_2).

Air is composed of a _____ of gases.

mixture

The two gases that primarily make up air are O_2 and _____.

N_2

Note: The total pressure exerted by the air is referred to as the *total atmospheric pressure* (P_{atm}). At sea level, it is about 760 mmHg. Atmospheric pressure varies with weather conditions and altitudes (i.e., above or below sea level). The higher the altitude, the lower the P_{atm}.

As you go higher above sea level, atmospheric pressure

_____.

decreases

$$PO_2 = FO_2 \times P_{atm}$$

To calculate the partial pressure of a gas in a mixture, take the fractional concentration of the gas and multiply it by the total atmospheric pressure.

We abbreviate the fractional concentration of any gas as FX, so the fractional concentration of O_2 is _____.

FO_2

We know that _____ percent of air is O_2, and this is called its fractional concentration.

21

The partial pressure of any gas in a mixture can be calculated if the total pressure of the mixture and fractional _____ of that gas are known.

concentration

To calculate the PO_2 of room air, we multiply 0.21×760 (i.e. $FO_2 \times P_{atm}$ to get _____ mmHg.

159

Since 79 percent of the atmosphere is N_2, the PN_2 is 79 percent of the total, or _____ mmHg (i.e., 79% of 760).

600

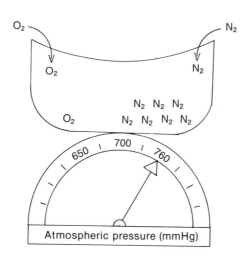

The O_2 and N_2 in air each contribute to the P_{atm} in proportion to their fractional concentration.

Air is mostly composed of O_2 and N_2, each with its own concentration and partial _____.

pressure

The total pressure of air is a sum of various partial pressures and equals _____.

760 mmHg

Note: This concept is summarized by Dalton's law of partial pressures. Its key elements include the following:

☐ The total pressure of a gas mixture is equal to the sum of the partial pressures of the gases in that mixture.
☐ The partial pressure exerted by each gas is proportional to its fractional percentage of the mixture.

Dalton's law is often expressed as: $P_1 + P_2 + P_3 + P_x = P_{total}$

In the case of atmospheric pressure,* $PO_2 + PN_2 = $ _____.

P_{atm}

*Assumes dry gas.

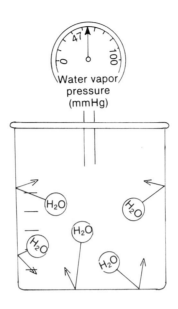

If water (H_2O) is present in vapor form in a gas mixture (i.e., humidity), it will exert its own partial pressure as will any other gas in the mixture.

Note: The amount of pressure exerted by water vapor depends on the relative humidity (RH) and temperature of the gas. Usually gas in alveoli is fully saturated with water vapor (100% RH) and has a partial pressure of water of 47 mmHg (i.e., PH_2O = 47 mmHg*).

Water vapor exerts a _____ when in a gas mixture.   *pressure*

PH_2O depends on both the RH and the _____ of the   *temperature*
gas.

Saturated gas at body temperature has a PH_2O of _____.   *47 mmHg*

Note: When describing gas that is inspired, the notation *I* is used. For example, the partial pressure of inspired O_2 is referred to as the PIO_2. The fractional concentration of inspired O_2 is FIO_2.
*Assumes body temperature of 37°C.

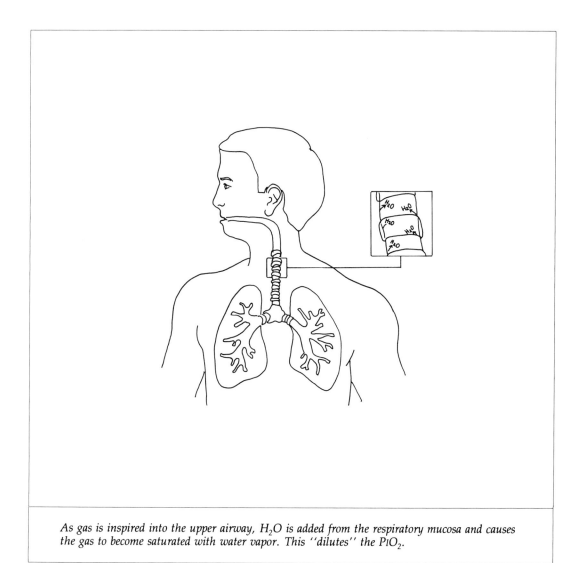

As gas is inspired into the upper airway, H₂O is added from the respiratory mucosa and causes the gas to become saturated with water vapor. This "dilutes" the PIO₂.

Gas inspired into the lungs has _____ vapor added to it in the upper airway.

water

The addition of water vapor _____ the PIO₂.

dilutes or reduces

Inspired gas is assumed to have a PH₂O of _____.

47 mmHg

Note: In determining the partial pressure of the inspired gas mixture, we must take into account the dilutional effect of PH₂O. This is achieved by calculating the total pressure available for all gases in the mixture and subtracting the PH₂O. This is referred to as the *dry* P$_{atm}$.

$$\text{dry } P_{atm} = (P_{atm} - PH_2O)$$

Atmospheric pressure corrected for the presence of water vapor is referred to as the dry P_{atm}.

Note: To accurately calculate partial pressures of gases in the atmosphere, we must correct for changes due to the presence of water vapor (i.e., humidity). This corrected P_{atm} is referred to as dry P_{atm}. It is this dry P_{atm} that we use when calculating the partial pressure of gases such as O_2 in inspired air.

Example: What would be the PIO_2 of a patient breathing room air?

$$PIO_2 = (\text{dry } P_{atm}) \, FIO_2$$
$$= (P_{atm} - PH_2O) \, FIO_2$$
$$= (760 - 47) \, 0.21$$
$$= 149 \text{ mmHg}$$

What would you calculate the PIN_2 to be? _____   *563 mm Hg*

(If you got that one right, you are really getting the hang of it!)

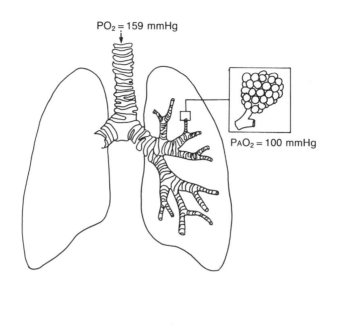

PO$_2$ = 159 mmHg

P$_A$O$_2$ = 100 mmHg

Although the PO$_2$ in the atmosphere is 159 mmHg, by the time O$_2$ reaches the alveoli it has decreased to about 100 mmHg.

The average PO$_2$ in the air we breathe is _____.

159 mmHg

Note: Remember, the P$_I$O$_2$ is reduced by the addition of PH$_2$O from the upper airway mucosa. Further dilution of the P$_I$O$_2$ occurs as the O$_2$ mixes with CO$_2$ present in the alveoli.

As O$_2$ is inspired into the lungs, the addition of water vapor and CO$_2$ causes the PO$_2$ to _____.

decrease

By the time O$_2$ reaches the lung alveoli, its partial pressure is about _____.

100 mmHg

Note: This is called the alveolar PO$_2$ and is expressed as P$_A$O$_2$.

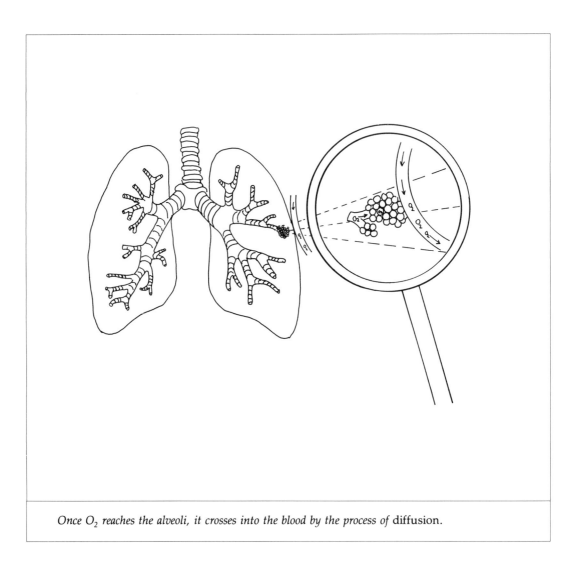

Once O_2 reaches the alveoli, it crosses into the blood by the process of diffusion.

Diffusion is the _____ of a gas from an area of high concentration (partial pressure) to one of lower concentration.

movement

Since the PO_2 is higher in the alveoli than in the venous capillary blood, O_2 will _____ into the blood.

diffuse

Note: There is further reduction in O_2 pressure as it diffuses through the alveolar walls on its way to the blood. The PO_2 in the arterial blood (PaO_2) averages 95 mmHg.

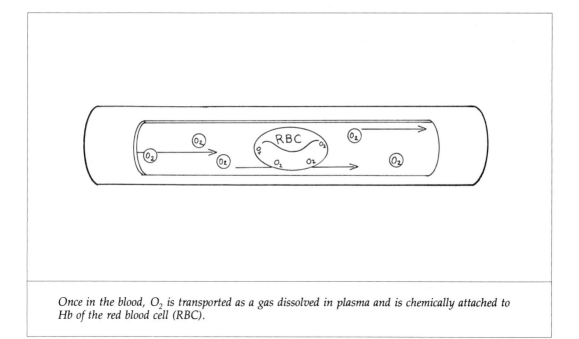

Once in the blood, O_2 is transported as a gas dissolved in plasma and is chemically attached to Hb of the red blood cell (RBC).

Note: Normally, 98 percent of O_2 in blood is transported attached to Hb, whereas only 2 percent is dissolved in plasma. However, this small amount of dissolved O_2 is quite important as it exerts the partial pressure responsible for the movement (diffusion) of O_2 into the tissues. It is the PO_2 exerted by this dissolved O_2 that is measured by an ABG.

Most of the O_2 entering the blood attaches to _____,
the major protein in the blood.

Hb

A small but significant portion of O_2 is dissolved in _____.

plasma

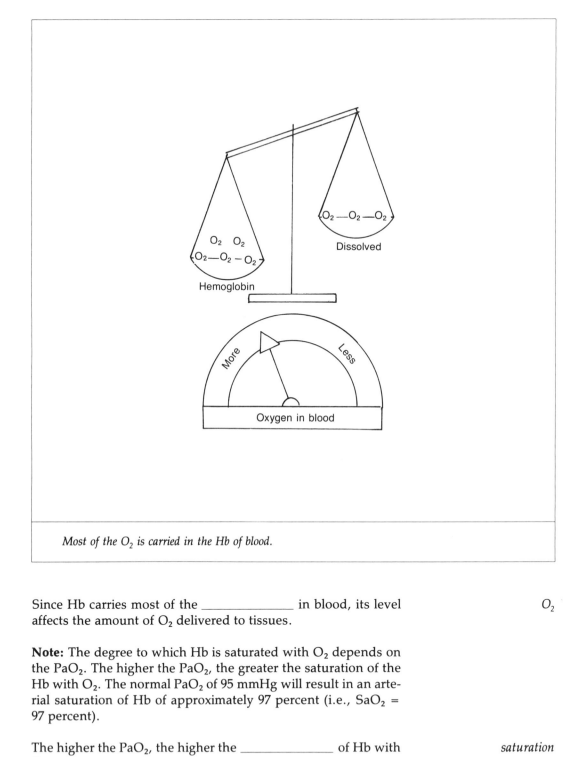

Most of the O_2 is carried in the Hb of blood.

Since Hb carries most of the _____ in blood, its level affects the amount of O_2 delivered to tissues.

O_2

Note: The degree to which Hb is saturated with O_2 depends on the PaO_2. The higher the PaO_2, the greater the saturation of the Hb with O_2. The normal PaO_2 of 95 mmHg will result in an arterial saturation of Hb of approximately 97 percent (i.e., SaO_2 = 97 percent).

The higher the PaO_2, the higher the _____ of Hb with O_2.

saturation

A PaO_2 of 95 mmHg will cause the SaO_2 to be _____ percent.

97

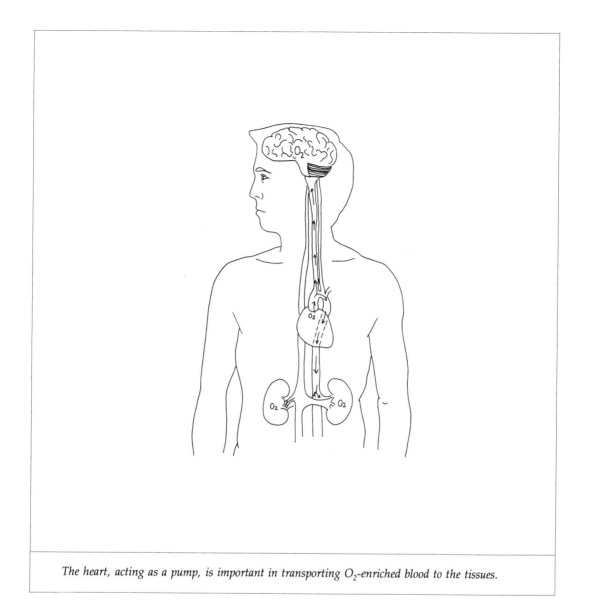

The heart, acting as a pump, is important in transporting O_2-enriched blood to the tissues.

An important factor in the transport of oxygenated blood to
_____ is the cardiac output.   *tissues*

The heart acts as a _____ and helps deliver blood to   *pump*
the tissues.

An ineffective output of blood by the heart will impair _____ O_2
delivery to the tissues.

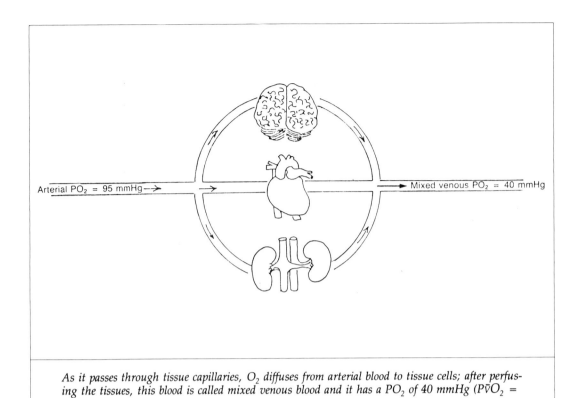

As it passes through tissue capillaries, O_2 diffuses from arterial blood to tissue cells; after perfusing the tissues, this blood is called mixed venous blood and it has a PO$_2$ of 40 mmHg ($P\bar{v}O_2$ = 40 mmHg).

Blood reaching the tissue capillaries has a PaO$_2$ of _____.

95 mmHg

Blood returning from perfused tissues is referred to as _____ venous blood.

mixed

The PO$_2$ in mixed venous blood is indicated by the symbol _____.

$P\bar{v}O_2$

Note: There is considerable variation in the consumption of O_2 by different organs. For example, the heart extracts almost all of the O_2 presented to it, whereas the skin utilizes very little. Since it is not practical to measure the PO$_2$ in venous blood returning from each individual organ, we usually measure the average in a representative sample of venous blood. This blood is obtained from the pulmonary artery by a special catheter (Swan-Ganz) that is usually reserved for monitoring critically ill patients.

The average PO$_2$ remaining after the tissues consume what they need is _____.

40 mmHg

Note: There is still a reserve of O_2 left after normal tissue extraction. Usually the Hb is 75 percent saturated with O_2 when it returns to the lungs ($S\bar{v}O_2$ = 75 %).

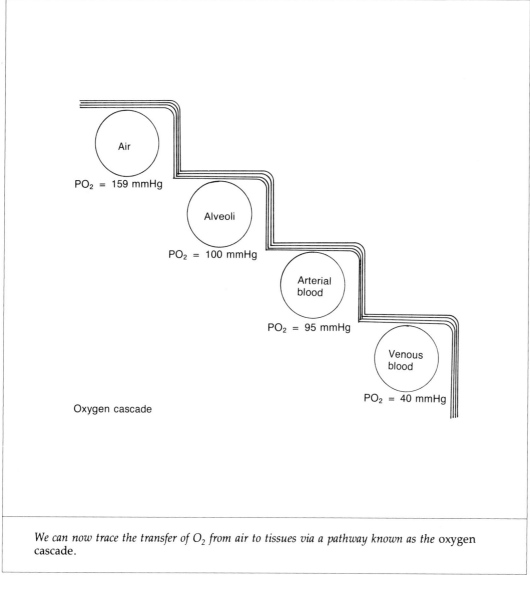

Air
$PO_2 = 159$ mmHg

Alveoli
$PO_2 = 100$ mmHg

Arterial blood
$PO_2 = 95$ mmHg

Venous blood
$PO_2 = 40$ mmHg

Oxygen cascade

We can now trace the transfer of O_2 from air to tissues via a pathway known as the oxygen cascade.

Although the PO_2 in air is _____, it is reduced to _____ when diluted by water vapor and CO_2 in the alveoli.

159 mmHg
100 mmHg

The PO_2 drops further as it diffuses from alveoli into the pulmonary capillary blood. The average PaO_2 is _____.

95 mmHg

As O_2 is consumed by tissue cells, the PO_2 _____ further.

falls

Venous blood returning from the tissues to the lungs has an average PO_2 value of _____.

40 mmHg

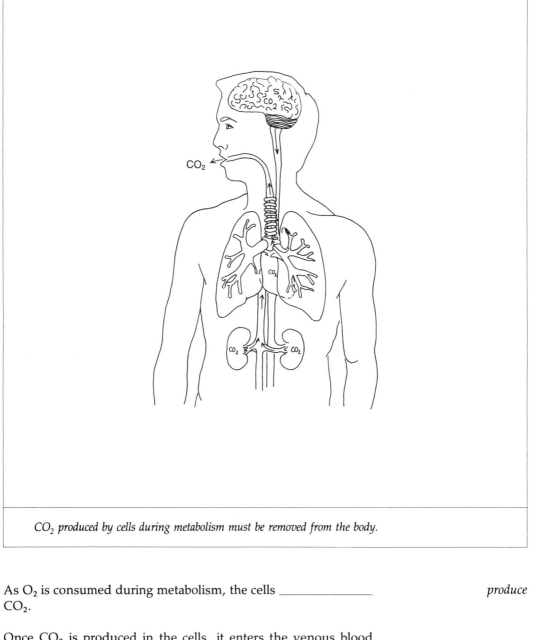

CO_2 produced by cells during metabolism must be removed from the body.

As O_2 is consumed during metabolism, the cells _____ *produce*
CO_2.

Once CO_2 is produced in the cells, it enters the venous blood
where it is transported to the _____ for removal. *lungs*

Note: The normal pressure of CO_2 in mixed venous blood is 46
mmHg (i.e., $P\bar{v}CO_2 = 46$ mmHg).

Once transported to the lungs, CO_2 is removed through the process of alveolar _____. *ventilation*

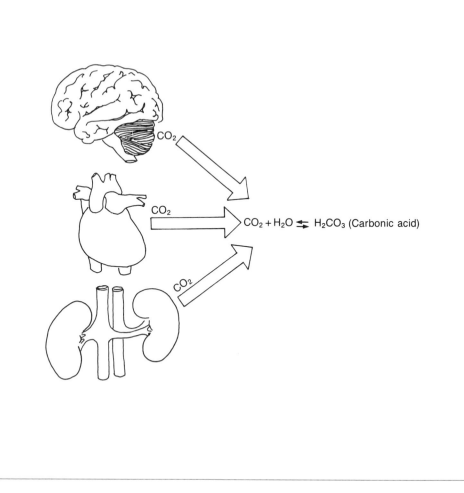

CO$_2$ produced during metabolism combines with H$_2$O to form a very important substance—carbonic acid (H$_2$CO$_3$).

CO$_2$ combines with water to form _____ _____.

carbonic acid

Note: Acids such as carbonic acid that can form a gas are referred to as *volatile acids.* This property allows carbonic acid produced in the body to be eliminated as CO$_2$ gas by alveolar ventilation.

H$_2$CO$_3$ can be eliminated from the body in the form of _____ gas.

CO$_2$

Through the process of alveolar ventilation, the lungs play a very important role in helping to maintain acid-base _____.

balance

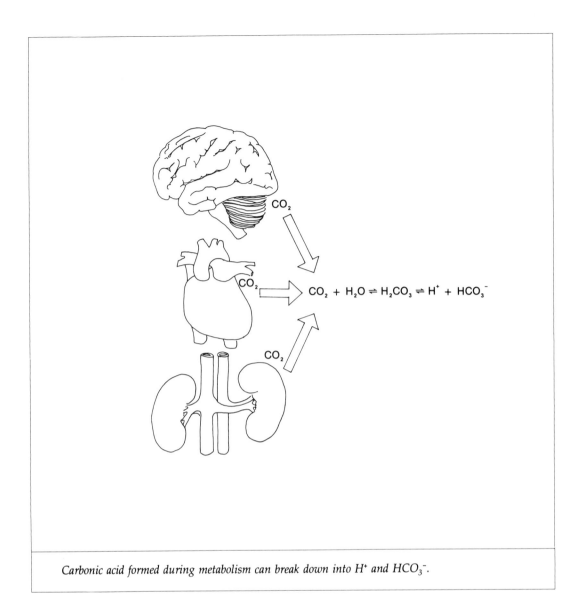

$$CO_2 + H_2O \rightleftharpoons H_2CO_3 \rightleftharpoons H^+ + HCO_3^-$$

Carbonic acid formed during metabolism can break down into H^+ and HCO_3^-.

H_2CO_3 is formed by combining CO_2 gas with _____. H_2O

Once H_2CO_3 is formed, it can break down into _____ H^+
and _____. HCO_3^-

Note: The ability of H_2CO_3 to donate H^+ to a solution makes it an acid (see Chap. 5).

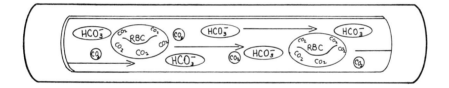

CO_2 is carried in the blood as HCO_3^-, attached to proteins (mostly Hb), and dissolved in plasma.

CO_2 is carried in the blood in _____ forms.

three

Note: About 5 percent of the CO_2 carried in the blood is dissolved in the plasma. Another 5 percent is chemically combined to proteins (mostly Hb). The vast majority of CO_2 (90%) is carried as HCO_3^-. This HCO_3^- is generated as follows:

$CO_2 + H_2O \rightleftharpoons H_2CO_3$, which dissociates into H^+ and HCO_3^-.

Most CO_2 is carried in the form of _____ ions.

HCO_3^-

In addition, CO_2 attaches to proteins and dissolves in _____.

plasma

Whereas most O_2 is carried in the blood attached to Hb, the majority of CO_2 is transported in the form of _____.

HCO_3^-

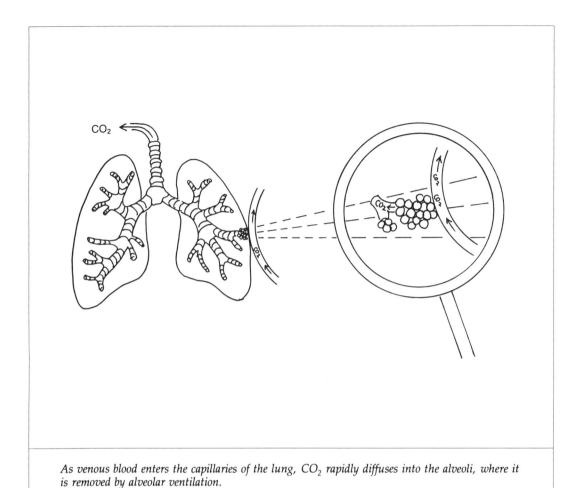

As venous blood enters the capillaries of the lung, CO_2 rapidly diffuses into the alveoli, where it is removed by alveolar ventilation.

Once venous blood is in the lung capillaries, CO_2 diffuses into the _____.

alveoli

Through the process of alveolar ventilation, CO_2 is _____ from the lungs.

removed

Note: We can see that the pressure of CO_2 in the arterial blood (i.e., $PaCO_2$) depends on the alveolar ventilation, which acts to "blow off" CO_2 and thereby control its value. The normal value for $PaCO_2$ is 40 mmHg. CO_2 can diffuse from venous blood to alveoli so easily that the arterial and alveolar values are usually considered the same ($PaCO_2 = PACO_2$).

By the time arterial blood leaves the lungs, its PCO_2 has dropped to _____.

40 mmHg

Note: Remember, it is the PCO_2 in *arterial* blood that is measured on an ABG.

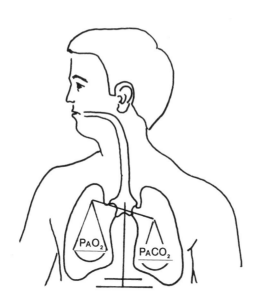

When breathing room air, there is a predictable relationship between alveolar O_2 and CO_2 levels (P_AO_2 and P_ACO_2).

Note: The total pressure of all gases in the alveoli must add up to atmospheric pressure. Therefore, as the partial pressure of one gas increases, the partial pressure of another must decrease. When breathing room air (21% O_2 and 79% N_2), there is a reciprocal relationship between the P_AO_2 and P_ACO_2. As one increases, the other must decrease and vice versa.

When breathing room air, there is a predictable relationship between the P_ACO_2 and the _____.

P_AO_2

When the P_ACO_2 increases, the P_AO_2 will _____.

decrease

When the P_ACO_2 decreases, the P_AO_2 will _____.

increase

Note: This rule of thumb is only applicable if the person is breathing room air. If the person is breathing an O_2-enriched mixture, this is not reliable. Also, keep in mind that this relationship pertains to the *alveolar* levels of O_2 and CO_2. Changes in alveolar PO_2 and PCO_2 do not always cause the same changes to occur in the *arterial* blood levels of PO_2 and PCO_2. (See Chap. 4.)

What is the *oxygenation* status?
What is the *ventilatory* status?
What is the *gas exchange* status?
What is the *acid-base* status?

When analyzing an ABG, we should always check these four general areas.

The _____ is used to determine the arterial oxygenation.

PaO₂

The PaCO₂ is used to evaluate the _____ status.

ventilatory

The combination of PaO₂ and PaCO₂ is used to evaluate

_____ _____ .

gas exchange

An evaluation of pH, PaCO₂, and HCO₃⁻ is used to determine
the _____ status.

acid-base

Bibliography

Boyce, B., and King, T. Blood gas and acid-base concepts in respiratory
care. *Am. J. Nurs.* 76 : 6, 1984.

Braun, H. A., Cheney, F., and Loehnen, P. *Introduction to Respiratory
Physiology* (2nd ed.). Boston: Little, Brown, 1980. Pp. 1–25.

Demers, R., and Saklad, M. Fundamentals of blood gas interpretation.
Resp. Care 78 : 2, 1973.

Flenley, D. Blood gas and acid-base interpretation. *Basics of RD, ATS
News,* Fall, 1981.

Golden, G., Litwiller, R., and Heironemus, T. The interpretation of arterial blood gases. *South. Med. J.* 66 : 9, 1973.

Harper, R. W. *A Guide to Respiratory Care: Physiology and Clinical Appli-
cations.* Philadelphia: Lippincott, 1982.

Lapuerta, L. *Blood Gases in Clinical Practice.* Springfield, Ill.: Thomas,
1976.

McPherson, S. P. *Respiratory Therapy Equipment* (2nd ed.). St. Louis:
Mosby, 1980.

Slonim, N. B., and Hamilton, L. H. *Respiratory Physiology* (5th ed.). St.
Louis: Mosby, 1987. Pp. 1–22.

Zagelbaum, G. L., and Pare, J. A. *Manual of Acute Respiratory Care.* Boston: Little, Brown, 1982.

2 The PaO₂

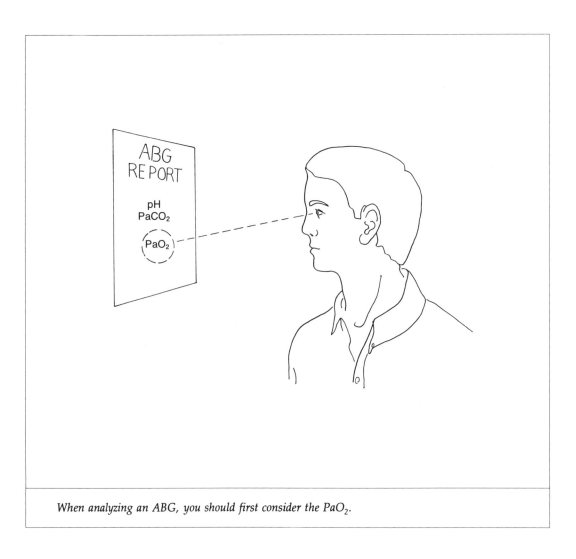

When analyzing an ABG, you should first consider the PaO_2.

O_2 dissolved in the blood exerts a _____ that can be measured.

pressure

A special electrode in a blood gas analyzer measures the PaO_2. This measurement is then reported on the _____ results.

ABG

When analyzing an ABG, arterial oxygenation is assessed by checking the _____.

PaO_2

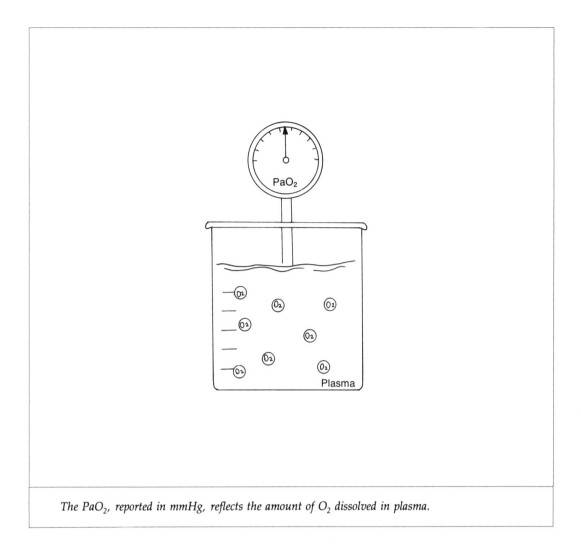

The PaO$_2$, reported in mmHg, reflects the amount of O$_2$ dissolved in plasma.

On an ABG report, the PaO$_2$ is reported in units of _____.　　　*mmHg*

The PaO$_2$ actually reflects the amount of O$_2$ dissolved in
_____.　　　*plasma*

Note: Since the source of blood for an ABG is an artery, the *a* is sometimes dropped. Thus, the PaO$_2$ is often referred to as the PO$_2$.

PaO$_2$ ≈ Arterial oxygenation

Although the PaO$_2$ actually reflects the amount of O$_2$ dissolved in the plasma, it is related to the total O$_2$ carried in the blood and can be used to provide a measure of arterial oxygenation.

The dissolved O$_2$ is related to the _____ O$_2$ carried in the blood.

total

The PaO$_2$ provides a measure of arterial _____.

oxygenation

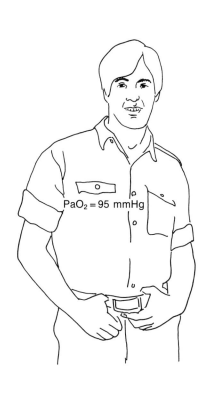

PaO₂ = 95 mmHg

The normal value for PaO₂ in young adults averages about 95 mmHg with a range of 85 to 100 mmHg.

The PaO₂ is usually within the range of _____.

85 to 100 mmHg

Even though the PO₂ of room air is 159 mmHg, by the time the O₂ reaches the arterial blood, the PaO₂ has dropped to an average value of _____.

95 mmHg

This drop in PO₂ from a room air level of 159 mmHg to an arterial blood level of 95 mmHg is primarily the result of the PO₂ being diluted with the addition of CO₂ gas and _____ vapor in the alveoli.

water

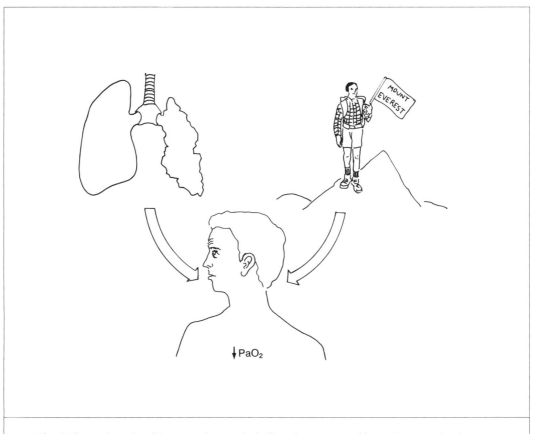

The PaO_2 can be reduced by many factors, including the presence of lung disease and a decrease in atmospheric pressure.

Although the normal PaO_2 is _____, this value can be affected by many factors.

95 mmHg

The PaO_2 can be lowered as a result of _____ disease.

lung

Even with healthy lungs, there are other factors that can reduce the PaO_2, such as breathing air with a low _____ pressure (e.g., high-altitude air).

atmospheric

Note: Some factors will actually *increase* PaO_2, such as giving a patient supplemental O_2 to breathe.

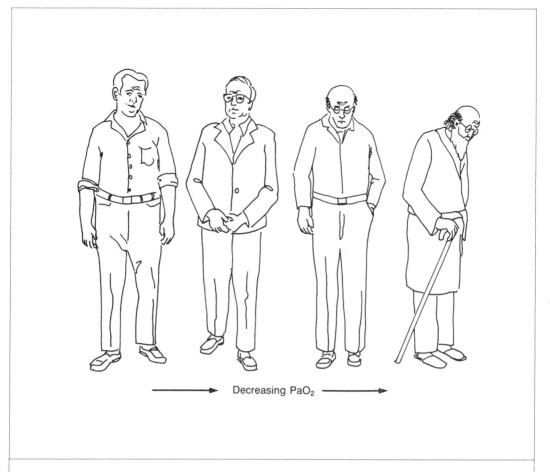

With advancing age, the normal value of PaO$_2$ falls steadily and averages about 80 mmHg at 60 years of age.

The normal aging process of the lungs results in changes that
_____ the PaO$_2$.

decrease

Note: As a general guideline, we can subtract 1 mmHg from a PaO$_2$ of 80 mmHg for every year over 60 years of age. Although this is only a rough rule of thumb, it provides an idea of what to anticipate in the older patient.

What is the lower limit of a normal expected PaO$_2$ in a 74-year-old patient? _____

66 mmHg

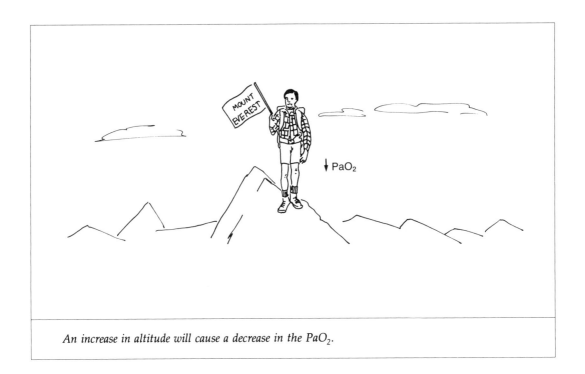

An increase in altitude will cause a decrease in the PaO$_2$.

Note: The O$_2$ concentration of air does not change with altitude. Air still has 21 percent O$_2$ even on the top of Mount Everest! What does decrease is the atmospheric (i.e., barometric) pressure. As a result, the PO$_2$ of air decreases with increasing altitude. (Remember: PO$_2$ = P$_{atm}$ × FO$_2$, which means that the PO$_2$ will decrease if P$_{atm}$ decreases.) In a person going from sea level to Denver, the level of PO$_2$ in the atmosphere falls from 150 mmHg to about 120 mmHg. High in the villages of the Andes, the PIO$_2$ may be as low as 70 mmHg and at the top of Mount Everest it is about 42 mmHg!

Although the fraction of inspired O$_2$ does not change with altitude, the _____ pressure does.

atmospheric

As atmospheric pressure falls, the PIO$_2$ decreases and this causes the PAO$_2$ to _____.

decrease

A decrease in PAO$_2$ will cause the PaO$_2$ to _____.

decrease

Note: To compensate for a lower PaO$_2$, people living at high altitudes increase their level of ventilation and may even develop variant Hb that allow their blood to carry more O$_2$!

The low cabin pressure in commercial airplanes (they are pressurized to the same atmospheric pressure that occurs at an altitude of 5000–8000 feet) can reduce the surrounding PO$_2$ enough to pose a threat to the passenger with significant lung disease.

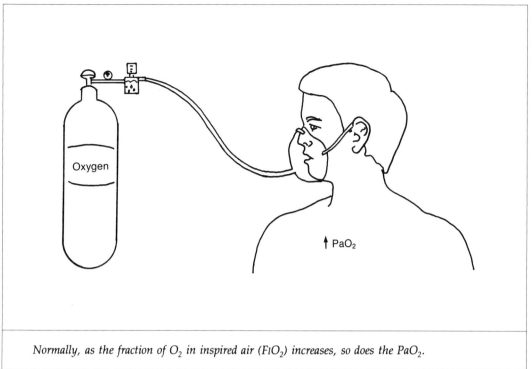

Normally, as the fraction of O_2 in inspired air (FiO$_2$) increases, so does the PaO$_2$.

We know that O_2 is normally _____ percent of room air.

21

Note: When the FiO$_2$ is increased (such as by giving an individual supplemental O_2 to breathe), the resulting rise in PaO$_2$ will cause the PaO$_2$ to increase. The amount it increases will depend on the condition of the patient's lungs. If there is no lung disease, the increase in PaO$_2$ and PaO$_2$ will be the same. If there is significant lung disease, the PaO$_2$ may not go up at all! A general rule of thumb is to multiply the FiO$_2$ by five to get a rough estimate of the expected PaO$_2$ for any particular level of inspired O_2. However, keep in mind that lung disease will often prevent the PaO$_2$ from rising as expected.

When O_2 is given to a patient, we are increasing the _____ that the patient is breathing.

FiO$_2$

An increase in FiO$_2$ *should* result in an increase in the _____.

PaO$_2$

What PaO$_2$ would you predict for a patient breathing an FiO$_2$ of 40%? _____

$\approx 200\ mmHg$

Note: If the PaO$_2$ is significantly less than predicted, it is often due to a gas-exchange problem caused by lung disease.

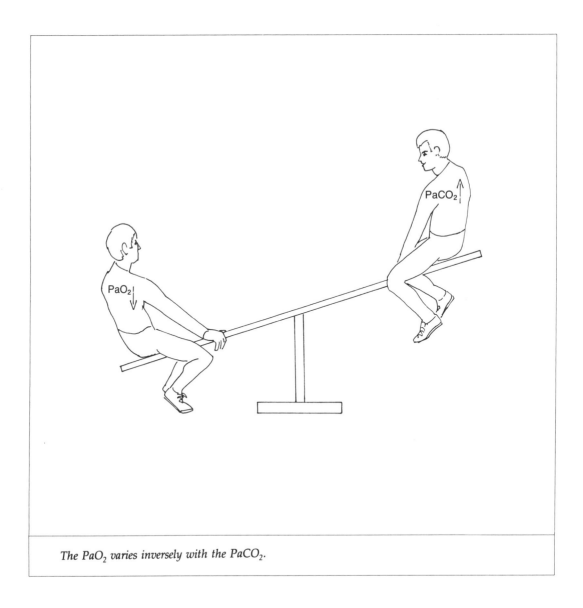

The PaO$_2$ varies inversely with the PaCO$_2$.

Note: The PaO$_2$ will usually vary with changes in alveolar ventilation. In general, when the PaCO$_2$ falls (i.e., ventilation is increased), the PaO$_2$ should rise by an equivalent amount. This is due to the reciprocal relationship between PACO$_2$ and PAO$_2$. When PACO$_2$ falls, the PAO$_2$ will increase (see p. 37, Chap. 1). A rise in the PAO$_2$ will cause the PaO$_2$ to increase.

When PACO$_2$ decreases, the PAO$_2$ _____.

An increase in the PAO$_2$ will cause the _____ to rise.

If there is a fall in the PaCO$_2$ and the PaO$_2$ does not increase as expected, we are probably dealing with a problem in _____ _____.

increases

PaO$_2$

gas exchange

48

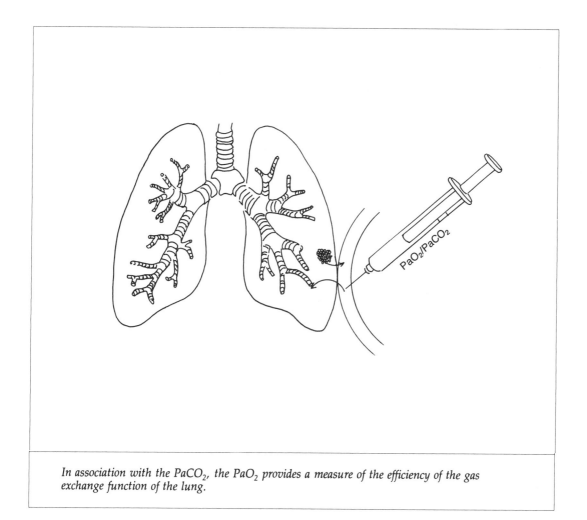

In association with the PaCO$_2$, the PaO$_2$ provides a measure of the efficiency of the gas exchange function of the lung.

A normal PaO$_2$ while breathing room air indicates that the transfer of _____ from the lungs to the blood is being accomplished effectively.

O$_2$

Note: If the measured PaO$_2$ while breathing room air is less than normal and supplemental O$_2$ is required to obtain a normal PaO$_2$, there is a gas exchange problem. This frequently occurs with lung disease and is suggested by the presence of an increased alveolar-to-arterial PO$_2$ gradient (A-aDO$_2$, see Chap. 4, pp. 121–129.)

If it takes an increased FIO$_2$ to achieve a normal PaO$_2$, the patient has a _____ problem.

gas exchange

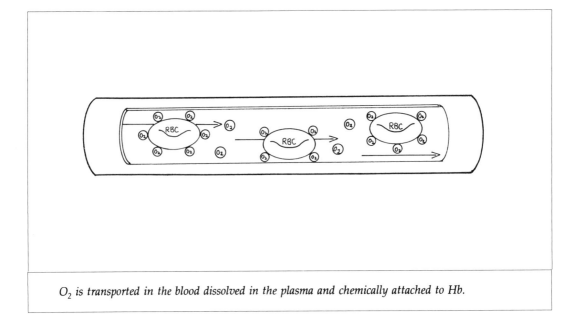

O_2 is transported in the blood dissolved in the plasma and chemically attached to Hb.

Once O_2 enters the blood, it dissolves in the _____.   *plasma*

Whereas some of the O_2 remains dissolved, most attaches to
_____ in the RBCs.   *Hb*

Note: Although the quantity of O_2 dissolved in the plasma is not large, the partial pressure exerted by this dissolved O_2 is responsible for the movement (diffusion) of O_2 from blood to the tissues.

$$O_2 \text{ dissolved in plasma} = (PaO_2) \times (0.003)$$

The quantity of O_2 dissolved in plasma is directly related to the PaO_2.

Note: For every 1 mmHg PaO_2, there will be 0.003 cc of O_2 dissolved in 1 dl of blood. This is shown by the following formula:

O_2 dissolved in plasma (cc/dl blood) = $(PaO_2) \times (0.003)$

For example: if the PaO_2 is 100 mmHg, how much O_2 would be dissolved in the plasma?

Answer: $(100) \times (0.003) = 0.3$ cc O_2/dl blood.

The quantity of O_2 dissolved in plasma is related to the level of
_____.

PaO_2

If the PaO_2 were to double, the amount of O_2 dissolved in the plasma would _____.

double

Note: Remember that 98% of O_2 carried in blood is attached to Hb. Therefore, even if we double or triple the amount of O_2 dissolved in plasma by giving the patient supplemental oxygen to breathe, this increased amount of transported O_2 is not significant when compared with the quantity that can be carried by the Hb.

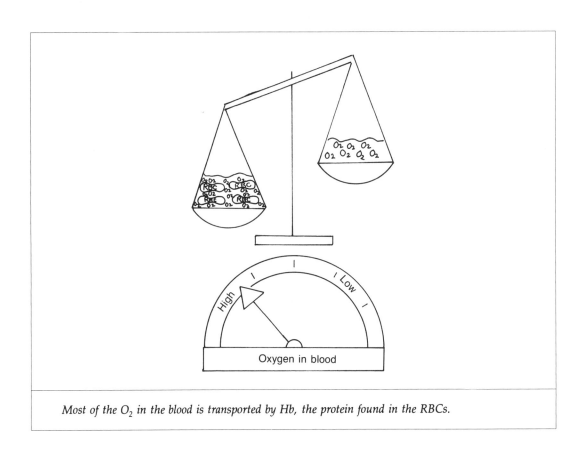

Most of the O_2 in the blood is transported by Hb, the protein found in the RBCs.

The total amount of O_2 carried in the blood depends largely on the _____ concentration, since the amount dissolved in plasma is quite small.

Hb

The Hb acts as a vehicle, picking up _____ in the pulmonary circulation and carrying it to the tissues.

O_2

As O_2 enters the blood, most of it attaches to the Hb, a _____ found in the RBCs.

protein

Note: Just how full or saturated with O_2 the Hb becomes will depend on the PO_2 of the blood and the chemical attractive forces between O_2 and Hb (i.e., their "affinity" for each other). When fully saturated, each gram of Hb can carry approximately 1.36 cc of O_2 (i.e., the oxygen-carrying capacity). In actuality, however, Hb does not usually carry its full complement of O_2, but the level is usually adequate to fill the needs of the tissues.

The presence of Hb markedly _____ the amount of O_2 that can be carried in the blood.

increases

Note: Hb that contains O_2 has a bright red appearance, whereas unoxygenated Hb is a dark blue color.

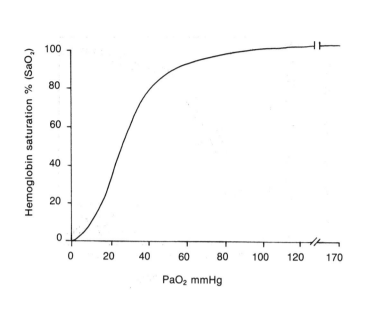

The saturation of Hb with O_2 will vary according to the level of PaO_2 and is expressed by a curve called the oxyhemoglobin dissociation curve.

The degree of saturation of Hb with O_2 will vary with the _____ in the plasma.

PO_2

As the PaO_2 increases, the _____ of Hb with O_2 will rise.

saturation

As the PaO_2 decreases, the saturation of Hb with O_2 _____.

falls

Note: Carefully study the general shape of the curve. Note the relatively steep portion of the curve at lower PaO_2s and the relatively flat portion at higher PaO_2s. This general shape is thought to be of physiologic importance. The steep portion of the curve indicates that a small drop in PaO_2 will cause a large drop in Hb saturation, thereby unloading large amounts of O_2 where needed (i.e., at the tissues). The flat portion tells us that the PaO_2 can fall a considerable amount and yet still maintain adequate arterial saturation. Hence, mild lung disease does not significantly interfere with oxygenation of the blood.

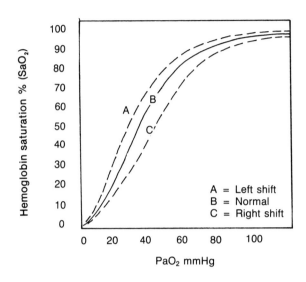

Y-axis: Hemoglobin saturation % (SaO₂)

X-axis: PaO₂ mmHg

A = Left shift
B = Normal
C = Right shift

Changes in the environment of the blood can change the affinity of Hb for O₂ and shift the oxy-hemoglobin curve toward the right or left.

A shift in the oxyhemoglobin curve indicates a change in the _____ of Hb for O₂.

affinity

Note: Since changes in affinity are primarily of theoretical rather than practical concern, we will only review a couple of the basic concepts.

A shift to the right means that a higher PaO_2 is needed to achieve the same Hb saturation than before the shift occurred. This is tantamount to a "decreased affinity." Conversely, a shift to the left means that a lower PaO_2 is needed to achieve the same Hb saturation than before the shift. This tells us that the affinity of Hb for O_2 is increased. Changes in the pH, $PaCO_2$, and temperature of the blood are factors that can change the affinity between Hb and O_2.

A shift of the curve to the _____ indicates a decrease in Hb and O₂ affinity.

right

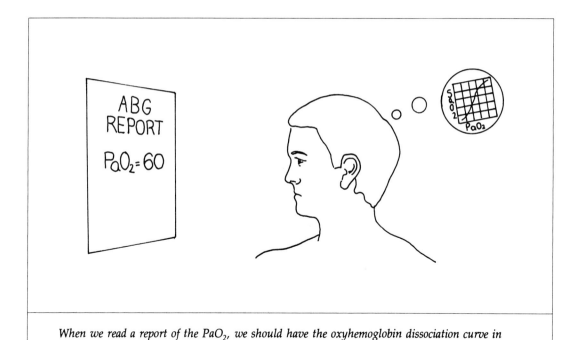

When we read a report of the PaO$_2$, we should have the oxyhemoglobin dissociation curve in mind.

Note: You have probably noted that the oxyhemoglobin dissociation curve is not linear. It is important to note that a PaO$_2$ of 60 mmHg represents close to 90 percent saturation of Hb with O$_2$ and that increasing the PaO$_2$ above 60 mmHg results in only a small increase in SaO$_2$. By observing the curve, we can also see that the PaO$_2$ must fall to 60 mmHg before significant desaturation of the Hb occurs (assuming normal affinity of Hb for O$_2$). A saturation of 90 percent or higher is usually considered adequate oxygenation of arterial blood. Remember that the total amount of O$_2$ carried in blood depends largely on the Hb concentration as well as the saturation.

From the oxyhemoglobin dissociation curve, we can see that a PaO$_2$ of 60 mmHg usually corresponds to an SaO$_2$ of _____ percent.

90

As the PaO$_2$ drops below 60 mmHg, the HbO$_2$ saturation falls _____.

rapidly

As the PaO$_2$ rises above 60 mmHg, the HbO$_2$ percent saturation increases _____.

slowly

Note: We can see that a patient with a PaO$_2$ below 60 mmHg is on the ''edge of a cliff'' and about to fall off. If the PaO$_2$ decreases by only a small amount, the corresponding decrease in SaO$_2$ can be disastrous!

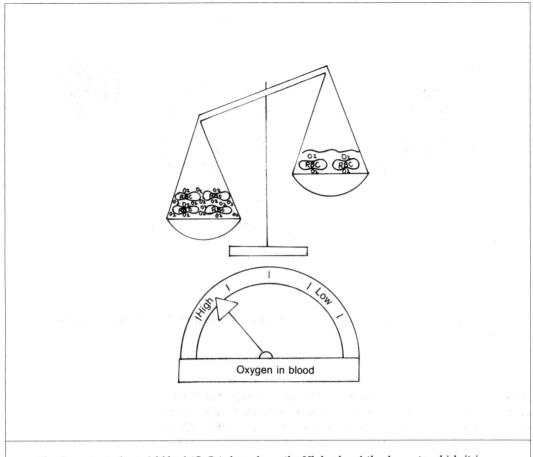

The O_2 content of arterial blood (CaO_2) depends on the Hb level and the degree to which it is saturated with O_2.

Arterial O_2 content refers to the total amount of O_2 carried in the arterial blood in all forms and is expressed by the symbol _____.

CaO_2

Note: CaO_2 is expressed in cc per dl of blood.

As Hb becomes more saturated with O_2, the O_2 content of blood _____.

increases

One of the main factors influencing the O_2 content of blood is the amount of _____ available to transport the O_2.

Hb

Since most of the O_2 is carried in Hb, anemia or acute blood loss will cause a _____ in CaO_2.

decrease

When the PaO_2 falls below 60 mmHg, the decrease in SaO_2 lowers the O_2 _____ of arterial blood.

content

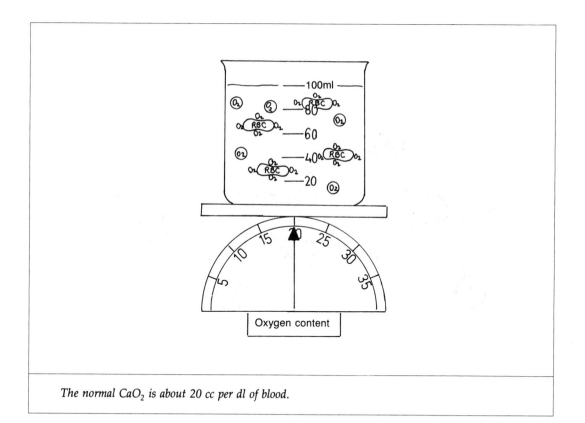

The normal CaO$_2$ is about 20 cc per dl of blood.

CaO$_2$ refers to the arterial blood O$_2$ _____.

content

The total CaO$_2$ is the sum of the O$_2$ _____ in plasma and that combined with Hb in the RBCs.

dissolved

Note: Each gram of Hb can carry 1.36 cc O$_2$ when fully saturated.

The total amount of O$_2$ carried by Hb will depend on the amount of Hb and the degree of _____ with O$_2$.

saturation

Note: We can calculate the CaO$_2$ as follows:

CaO$_2$ = O$_2$ combined with Hb + dissolved O$_2$ in plasma

O$_2$ combined with Hb = gm Hb × saturation of Hb × 1.36, if

Hb = 15 and PaO$_2$ = 90 (i.e., SaO$_2$ = 97%)

O$_2$ combined with Hb = 15 × 0.97 × 1.36

$$= 19.79 \text{ cc}$$

Dissolved O$_2$ in plasma = 90 × 0.003

Therefore CaO$_2$ = 19.79 + 0.270 cc = 20.06 cc/dl

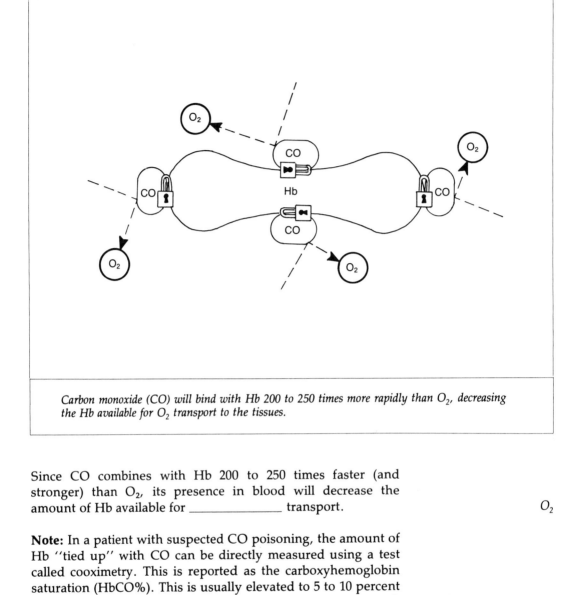

Carbon monoxide (CO) will bind with Hb 200 to 250 times more rapidly than O_2, decreasing the Hb available for O_2 transport to the tissues.

Since CO combines with Hb 200 to 250 times faster (and stronger) than O_2, its presence in blood will decrease the amount of Hb available for _____ transport.

O_2

Note: In a patient with suspected CO poisoning, the amount of Hb "tied up" with CO can be directly measured using a test called cooximetry. This is reported as the carboxyhemoglobin saturation (HbCO%). This is usually elevated to 5 to 10 percent in heavy smokers, and in smoke-inhalation victims may reach life-threatening levels of greater than 30 to 40 percent.

A person may have a normal PaO_2 but the _____ may be decreased by the presence of _____.

CaO_2
CO

CO may impair O_2 transport to the _____.

tissues

```
                PaO₂ < normal = Hypoxemia
```

A decrease in PaO₂ is a common finding in patients with lung disease and is called hypoxemia.

Hypoxemia refers to a decrease in _____ and is diagnosed by using an ABG.

Note: The severity of hypoxemia can be categorized according to
the following guidelines:

1. *Mild* hypoxemia is defined by a PaO₂ between 60 and 80
   mmHg.
2. *Moderate* hypoxemia is defined by a PaO₂ in the range of 40 to
   60 mmHg.
3. *Severe* hypoxemia is present when the PaO₂ falls below 40
   mmHg.

Review the above carefully. These descriptive terms are often
used when interpreting the arterial oxygenation status of an
ABG.

PaO₂

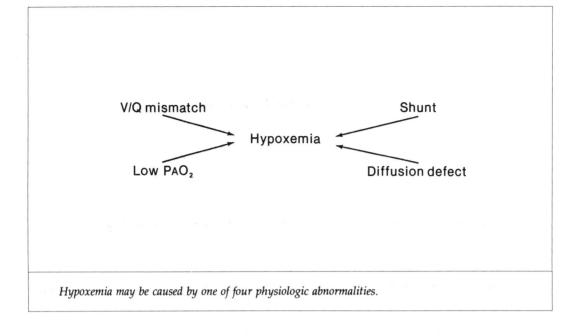

Hypoxemia may be caused by one of four physiologic abnormalities.

These are the four physiologic causes of hypoxemia:

1. Unequal matching of ventilation (V) to blood perfusion (Q) in the lungs (i.e., so-called V/Q mismatch). The specific type of mismatch that can result in hypoxemia is a decrease in ventilation relative to the amount of perfusion.
2. Shunting, the movement of blood from the right side of the heart to the left side of the heart without passing through the lungs; or blood passing through the lungs without any exposure to the alveolar gas (intrapulmonary shunt).
3. Low alveolar O_2 tension (decreased PAO_2) most commonly due to:
   a. A decrease in ventilation causing an increase in $PACO_2$ and $PaCO_2$ (hypoventilation)
   b. A drop in the level of inspired O_2 (breathing less than 21% O_2)
   c. Low P_{atm} causing the partial pressures of all gases to be low (breathing air at a high altitude)
4. An inability of O_2 to diffuse from the lung through the alveolar-capillary membrane and into the blood. This is referred to as a *diffusion defect.*

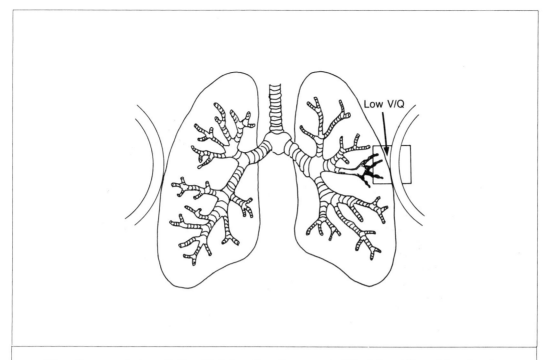

When the amount of ventilation (V) is less than the amount of blood flow (Q) reaching the alveoli, a decrease in the PaO_2 may result. This is known as a ventilation-perfusion (V/Q) mismatch.

Note: Normally, V/Q ratios of the lung average about 1 : 1. Lung diseases frequently result in an unequal distribution of inspired gas, causing a decrease in ventilation relative to perfusion. This is the most common cause of hypoxemia.

Ventilation is represented by the symbol _____.

V

The symbol Q is used to represent blood flow reaching the _____.

alveoli

A decrease in V in relation to Q (low V/Q) will cause the PaO_2 to _____.

decrease

A ventilation-perfusion or V/Q mismatch is the most common cause of _____.

hypoxemia

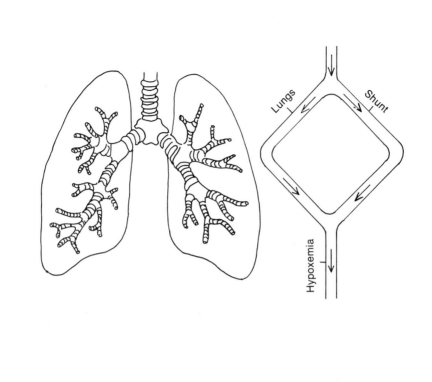

Venous blood that enters the arterial system without going through ventilated areas of lung is called shunted *blood and results in hypoxemia.*

Shunted blood is blood that goes from veins to arteries without passing through _____ areas of lung.

ventilated

Shunting will cause hypoxemia because the shunted venous blood entering arteries bypasses the lung and does not become replenished with _____.

O_2

Note: Hypoxemia caused by a shunt *does not* respond very well to O_2 therapy. In shunted areas, the venous blood bypasses the gas exchanging portions of lung. Consequently, breathing an increased FIO_2 will not result in additional O_2 being added to this blood.

The hallmark of a shunt is a failure of the PaO_2 to respond to large increases in the inspired _____ concentration.

O_2

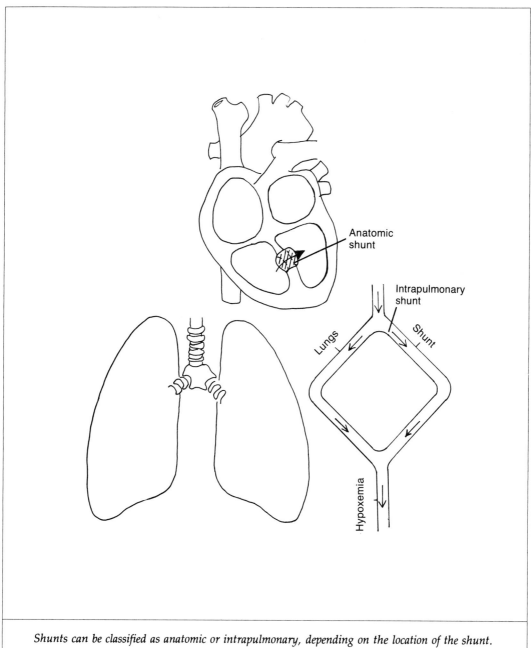

Shunts can be classified as anatomic or intrapulmonary, depending on the location of the shunt.

Blood that goes through abnormal anatomic communications (e.g., cardiac defects) and bypasses the lungs completely will result in an _____ shunt.

anatomic

Blood passing by collapsed alveoli (e.g., atelectasis) or fluid-filled alveoli (e.g., pneumonia or edema) causes _____ shunting.

intrapulmonary

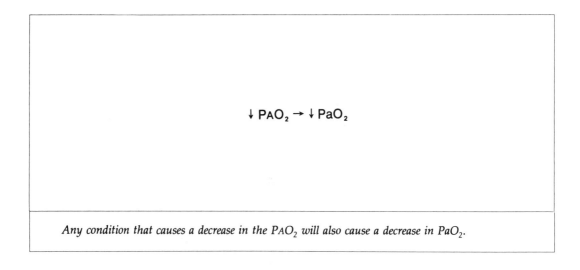

$$\downarrow PAO_2 \rightarrow \downarrow PaO_2$$

Any condition that causes a decrease in the PAO_2 will also cause a decrease in PaO_2.

Note: Normally, the pressure of O_2 in the pulmonary-capillary blood equilibrates with the pressure of O_2 in the alveoli. As a result, if the PAO_2 falls, the capillary blood PO_2 should fall by a proportionate amount.

A decrease in PAO_2 will result in a _____ in PaO_2.

decrease

Note: Common causes of a low PAO_2 include the following:

1. A decrease in ventilation causing an increase in $PACO_2$ and $PaCO_2$ (hypoventilation)
2. A drop in the level of inspired O_2 (i.e., breathing less than 21% O_2)
3. A low P_{atm} causing the partial pressures of all gases to be low (e.g., breathing air at a high altitude)

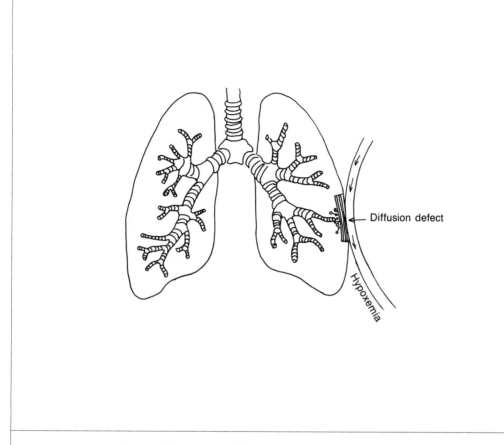

Any impairment in the ability of O_2 to diffuse from the lungs into the blood may result in hypoxemia.

An increased thickness of the alveolar-capillary membrane may impair O_2 diffusion and result in _____.

hypoxemia

A loss in surface area of lung tissue (e.g., as in emphysema) may decrease the amount of O_2 that _____ into the blood, resulting in hypoxemia.

diffuses

If the RBCs move through the lungs too quickly (as occurs during exercise when cardiac output is increased), there may be inadequate *time* for O_2 to _____ into the blood.

diffuse

Note: Diffusion defects *do not* usually affect CO_2 elimination since this gas diffuses 20 times more readily than O_2 through the alveolar-capillary membrane. When CO_2 elimination is impaired, it is almost always the result of inadequate alveolar ventilation.

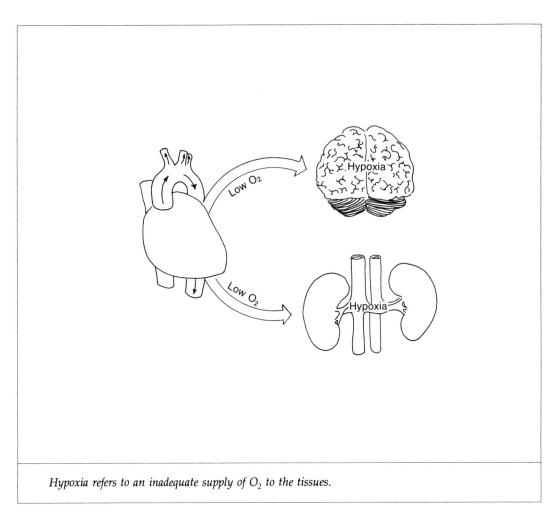

Hypoxia refers to an inadequate supply of O_2 to the tissues.

Hypoxemia is recognized by a low _____.

PaO_2

Hypoxia, on the other hand, refers to an inadequate supply of O_2 to the _____.

tissues

Hypoxemia poses a danger to the patient when it results in impaired tissue oxygenation, or _____.

hypoxia

Note: Hypoxemia is only one cause of hypoxia. A decrease in cardiac output and Hb deficiencies may also cause hypoxia by reducing the amount of O_2 delivered to the tissues.

The amount of _____ delivered to tissues depends on the cardiac output and the CaO_2.

O_2

Note: Hypoxia can also be caused by an inability of tissues to utilize available O_2. This can occur in cellular poisoning (e.g., cyanide poisoning).

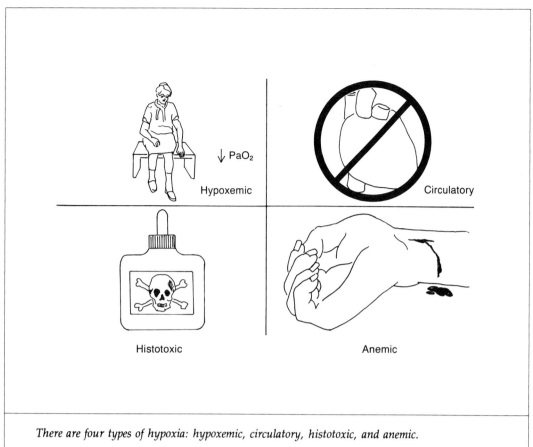

There are four types of hypoxia: hypoxemic, circulatory, histotoxic, and anemic.

If hypoxemia is severe and significantly lowers the CaO_2, this may also reduce tissue O_2 levels and is called hypoxemic

_____.   *hypoxia*

A decrease in cardiac _____ that results in hypoxia is   *output*
referred to as circulatory or stagnant hypoxia.

Reduced levels of Hb will lower the _____ content of O_2
the blood and, if severe, can cause anemic hypoxia.

If cells have been ''poisoned'' (e.g., with cyanide) and are unable to utilize O_2, the condition is referred to as histotoxic

_____.   *hypoxia*

Remember: Hypoxemia refers to a low PaO_2 and hypoxia to a
low tissue O_2 level.

Note: Hypoxemia is easy to diagnose. Just look at the PaO_2!
Hypoxia is more difficult to recognize and is usually suspected
on the basis of certain clinical findings (see p. 71).

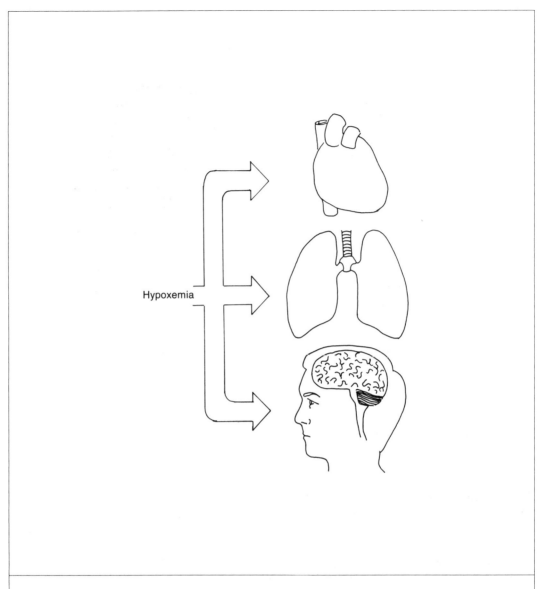

Hypoxemia

The signs and symptoms of hypoxemia are nonspecific and usually involve the cardiac, respiratory, and central nervous systems.

It is sometimes difficult to recognize the signs and symptoms of hypoxemia because they are _____.

nonspecific

Name the three major organ systems usually involved in the body's response to hypoxemia:

1. _____
2. _____
3. _____

cardiac
respiratory
central nervous

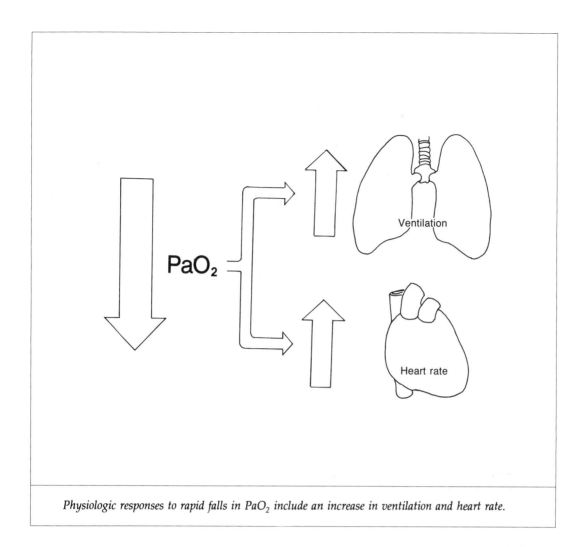

Physiologic responses to rapid falls in PaO$_2$ include an increase in ventilation and heart rate.

Sudden drops in PaO$_2$ cause _____ responses.

physiologic

By increasing ventilation, more _____ becomes available for diffusion into the arterial blood.

O$_2$

As our heart rate increases (i.e., tachycardia), the associated increase in cardiac output provides more blood and _____ to the tissues.

O$_2$

By increasing ventilation and cardiac output, more O$_2$ can be made available to the _____.

tissues

Note: In an attempt to compensate for any loss in the O$_2$-carrying capacity of the blood, the cardiac output and respiratory rate increase. These changes are associated with signs reflecting an increase in the work of breathing (e.g., tachypnea) and in the cardiac work (e.g., tachycardia).

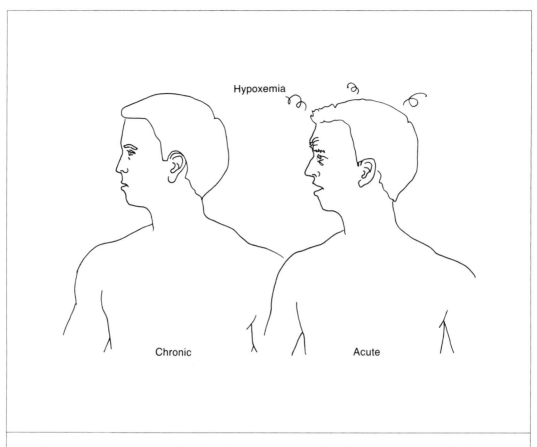

Hypoxemia of gradual onset (i.e., chronic) causes fewer clinical disturbances than rapidly developing hypoxemia (i.e., acute) even if the overall reduction in PaO₂ is the same.

Responses to chronic hypoxemia are usually less dramatic than those that occur in response to hypoxemia of _____ onset.

acute

Both acute and chronic physiologic responses are part of the body's attempt to compensate for a _____ of O_2.

lack

In response to hypoxemia of gradual onset, the production of RBCs is increased in an attempt to raise the _____ carrying capacity of blood.

O_2

Gradually developing hypoxemia is much better tolerated than that of _____ onset.

acute

Note: Another physiologic response to chronic hypoxemia is a decrease in the oxyhemoglobin affinity. This promotes easier release of O_2 to tissues by increasing the production of an enzyme (2,3-diphosphoglycerate) that shifts the oxyhemoglobin curve to the right.

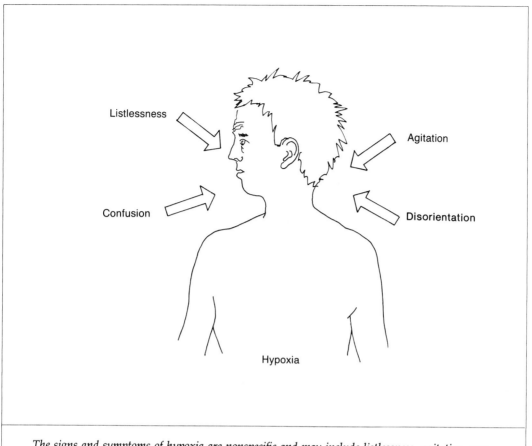

The signs and symptoms of hypoxia are nonspecific and may include listlessness, agitation, confusion, and disorientation.

A lack of adequate supply of _____ to the brain (cerebral hypoxia) can lead to various neurologic disturbances.

O_2

Changes in mentation such as agitation, confusion, and disorientation can be clinical clues to the presence of _____.

hypoxia

Note: When these findings occur in association with severe hypoxemia, they usually reflect cerebral hypoxia.

Unfortunately, the clinical findings of hypoxia are _____.

nonspecific

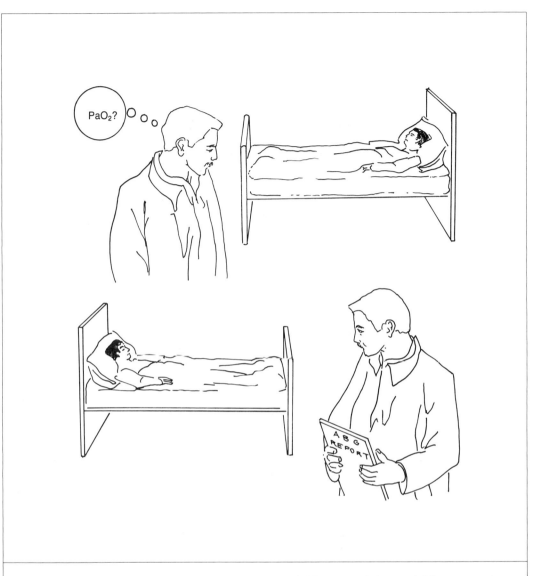

The clinical diagnosis of hypoxemia is notoriously unreliable. An ABG is essential for an accurate diagnosis.

The clinical diagnosis of hypoxemia is notoriously _____.   *unreliable*

Increases in the resting respiratory and heart rates are sensitive but nonspecific signs of _____.   *hypoxemia*

Although nonspecific, findings such as agitation, listlessness, and confusion *may* suggest the presence of _____.   *hypoxia*

To accurately diagnose hypoxemia, we must rely on an _____.   *ABG*

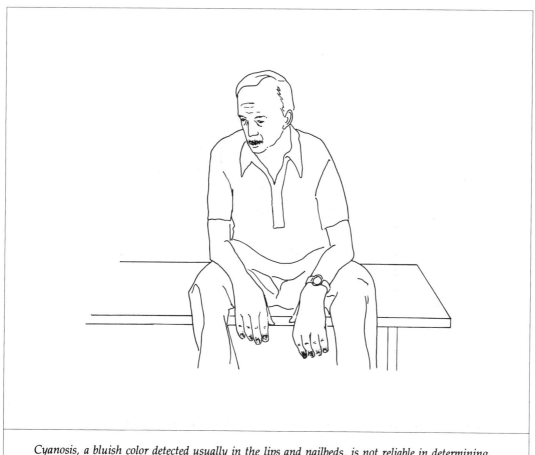

Cyanosis, a bluish color detected usually in the lips and nailbeds, is not reliable in determining the presence of hypoxemia.

The presence of 5 gm of unoxygenated Hb per dl of blood may result in a bluish color of mucous membranes known as

_____.

cyanosis

Lighting conditions, a patient's skin color, and Hb levels alter our ability to detect cyanosis, making it an _____ guide to the presence of hypoxemia.

unreliable

Note: The *sudden* appearance of cyanosis is, of course, a serious finding and warrants immediate attention. The presence of central cyanosis (i.e., cyanosis of the lips and mucous membranes) indicates a drop in O_2 saturation to approximately 80 percent of normal. Peripheral cyanosis (i.e., cyanosis of the extremities and nailbeds only) is less reliable and may reflect a local disorder due to impaired circulation.

One must not rely on the presence of cyanosis for the diagnosis of _____.

hypoxemia

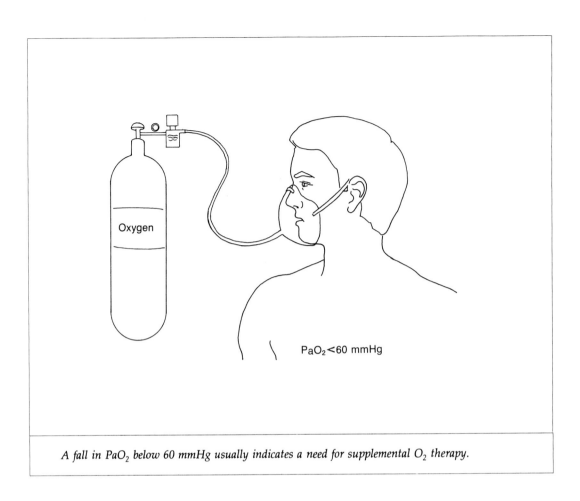

A fall in PaO₂ below 60 mmHg usually indicates a need for supplemental O₂ therapy.

As the PaO₂ falls below _____, the SaO₂ begins to fall rapidly.

60 mmHg

Thus, we usually treat a PaO₂ below 60 mmHg with supplemental _____ therapy.

O₂

Any drop in PaO₂ below 60 mmHg results in marked _____ of Hb with O₂.

desaturation

When the PaO₂ is above 60 mmHg (corresponding to an SaO₂ ≥ 90%), it is usually *not* necessary or therapeutic to administer _____.

O₂

Note: In patients with a reduced Hb, stroke, or a heart attack, however, higher levels of PaO₂ (≈ 100 mmHg) are considered desirable.

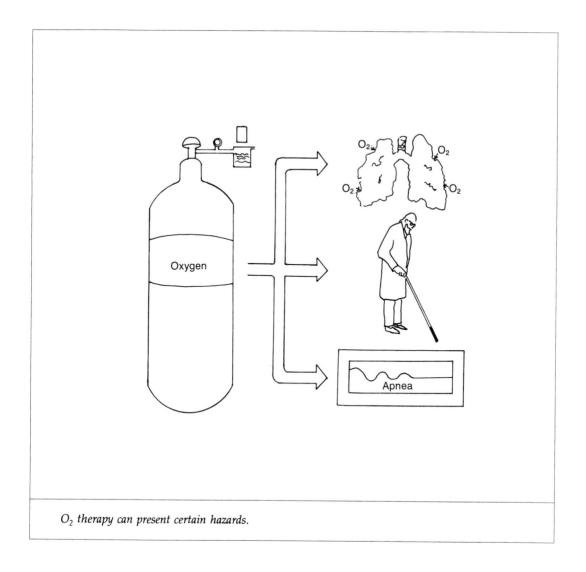

O_2 therapy can present certain hazards.

Although sometimes necessary, the administration of O_2 has
certain _____ .

hazards

Note: The hazards of O_2 administration are usually classified into three areas:

1. An FIO_2 over 50 percent for more than 24 hours *may* result in
   direct damage to the lung tissue referred to as *pulmonary oxygen toxicity.*
2. An elevated PaO_2 in the premature newborn *may* result in
   permanent damage to the retina of the eyes (retrolental
   fibroplasia or retinopathy of prematurity).
3. Patients with severe chronic obstructive lung disease and CO_2
   retention *may* have their ventilatory stimulus reduced by excessive correction of hypoxemia. This can lead to increasing
   CO_2 retention, acidemia, and clinical deterioration.

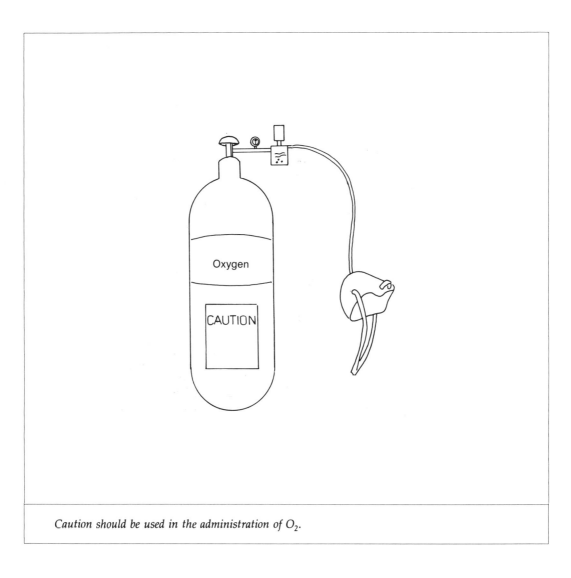

Caution should be used in the administration of O₂.

An FIO₂ over _____ for prolonged periods of time may result in _____ to the lungs.

50 percent
toxicity

A high PaO₂ in premature newborns may result in permanent damage to the retina of the _____.

eyes

Patients with chronic obstructive lung disease who receive excessive O₂ therapy may have their hypoxic ventilatory drive _____ by overcorrecting the PaO₂.

suppressed

Note: The golden rule is to treat O₂ as any other drug: use as little as possible and only for as long as is medically required.

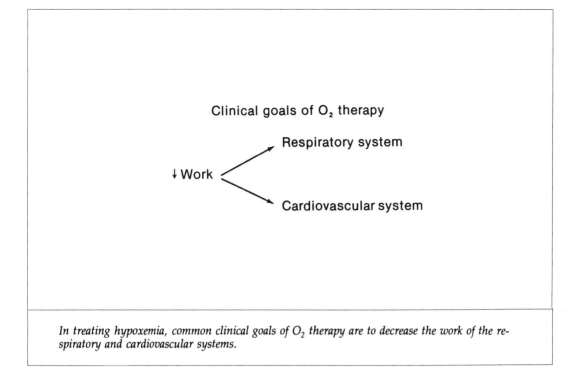

Clinical goals of O₂ therapy

↓ Work → Respiratory system
↓ Work → Cardiovascular system

In treating hypoxemia, common clinical goals of O_2 therapy are to decrease the work of the respiratory and cardiovascular systems.

An increase in the work of breathing often accompanies
_____ and is suggested by the presence of tachypnea.

hypoxemia

Note: In the presence of hypoxemia, a sensitive indicator of increased work of breathing is the patient's subjective complaint of feeling short of breath. This is referred to as *dyspnea*.

A patient who complains of feeling short of breath is said to be experiencing _____.

dyspnea

The tachycardia often seen in response to hypoxemia reflects an increase in the work of the _____ system.

cardiovascular

Bibliography

D'Alonzo, G. and Gutierrez, G. How to make sure oxygen delivery and consumption are adequate. *J of Resp Diseases*, October, 1985.

Fulmer, J., and Snider, G. ACCP-NHLBI national conference on oxygen therapy. *Chest* 86 : 2, 1984.

Kettel, L., et al. Recommendations for continuous oxygen therapy in chronic obstructive lung disease. *Chest* 64 : 4, 1973.

Shapiro, B. A., Harrison, R. A., and Walton, J. R. *Clinical Application of Blood Gases* (3rd ed.). Chicago: Year Book, 1982.

3 The PaCO$_2$

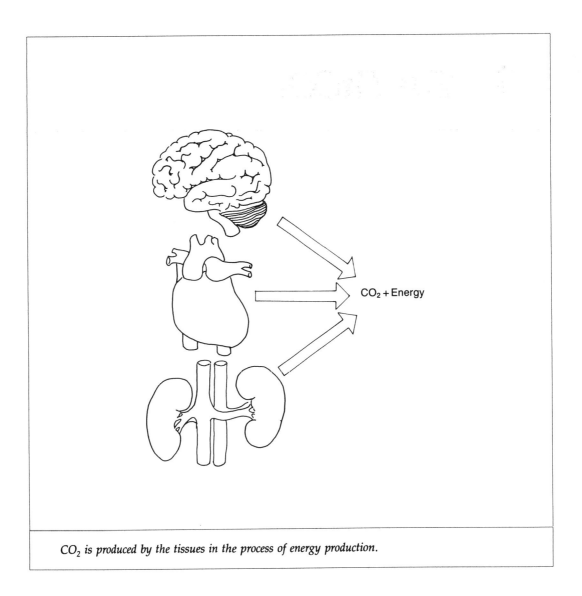

CO_2 + Energy

CO_2 is produced by the tissues in the process of energy production.

CO_2 is produced in the _____ as a result of metabolism.

tissues

During energy production by the tissues, O_2 is consumed and CO_2 is _____.

produced

Note: Under normal conditions, the tissues produce approximately 200 cc of CO_2 gas each minute. This gas must be eliminated efficiently or it will rapidly build up in the body.

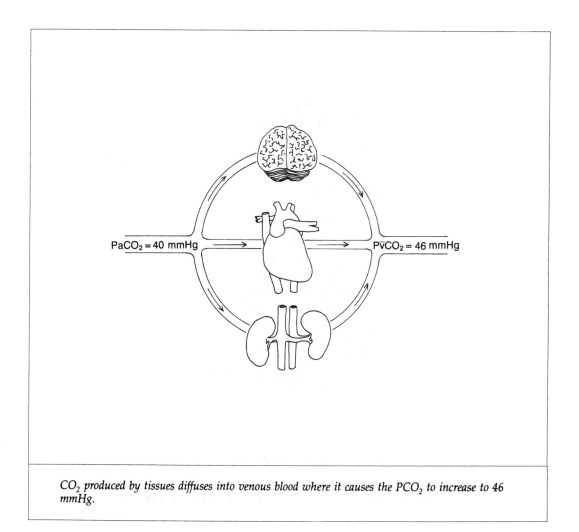

$PaCO_2 = 40$ mmHg $P\bar{v}CO_2 = 46$ mmHg

CO₂ produced by tissues diffuses into venous blood where it causes the PCO_2 to increase to 46 mmHg.

CO_2 diffuses from tissues into _____ blood.   *venous*

Note: To express the PCO_2 in *venous* blood, we use the letter *v*.
The bar over the *v* ($\bar{v}$) is necessary to indicate that the sample is
an average of venous blood from all parts of the body.

The normal $PaCO_2$ reaching the tissues is _____ .   *40 mmHg*

The normal $P\bar{v}CO_2$ leaving the tissues is _____ .   *46 mmHg*

81

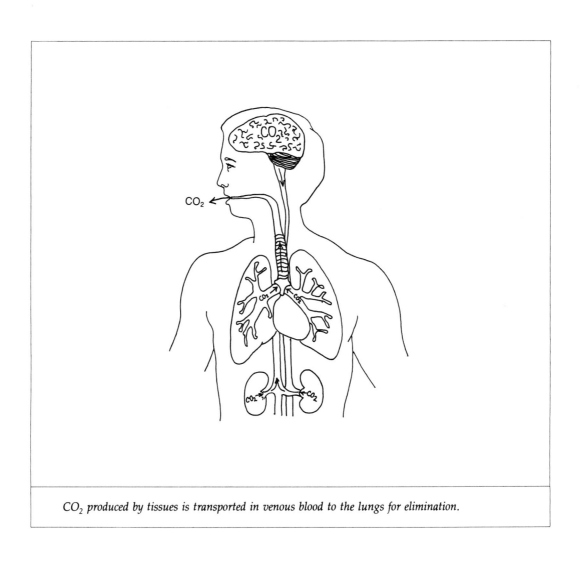

CO$_2$ *produced by tissues is transported in venous blood to the lungs for elimination.*

CO$_2$ produced by tissues during metabolism is transported to the lungs by _____ blood.

venous

In the lungs, CO$_2$ that was added at the tissues is _____ .

eliminated

Note: Once in the lungs, CO$_2$ *diffuses* from the blood into the alveoli where its partial pressure is 40 mmHg (P$_A$CO$_2$). Some of the CO$_2$ in the alveoli is then expired into the air with each breath. Of course, not all the CO$_2$ is eliminated. Even after a normal expiration, there is still a residual amount left in the alveoli that keeps the P$_A$CO$_2$ equal to 40 mmHg.

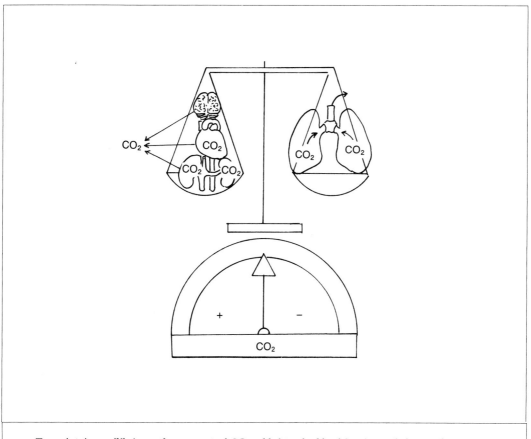

To maintain equilibrium, the amount of CO_2 added to the blood by tissues balances the amount eliminated by the lungs.

CO_2 is _____ to the blood by the tissues. *added*

CO_2 is _____ by the lungs. *eliminated*

Normally, the amounts of CO_2 produced and eliminated are maintained in _____. *equilibrium*

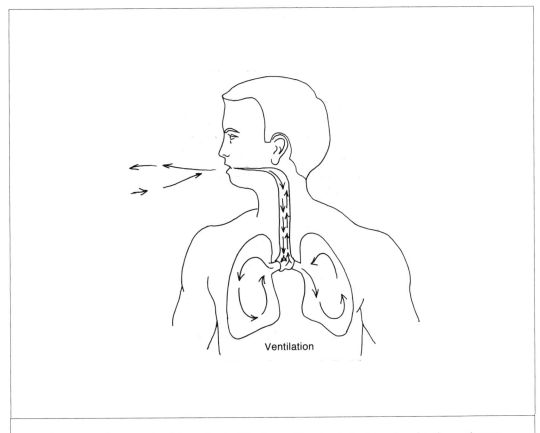

The process of gas moving into and out of the lungs (i.e., breathing) is referred to in respiratory physiology as ventilation.

Gas movement in and out of the lungs is referred to as

_____.

ventilation

Note: The amount of gas exhaled with each breath is referred to as the *tidal volume* (VT) and is approximately 500 ml in the average adult. The total amount of gas exhaled from the lungs in 1 minute is called *minute ventilation* ($\dot{V}$E). Minute ventilation can be calculated by multiplying the tidal volume by the frequency of ventilations (f). For example, if the respiratory frequency is 12 per minute, the normal minute volume can be calculated as follows:

$$\dot{V}E \ = \ VT \times f \ = \ (500 \ ml)(12) \ = \ 6000 \ ml/min \text{ or } 6 \ L/min$$

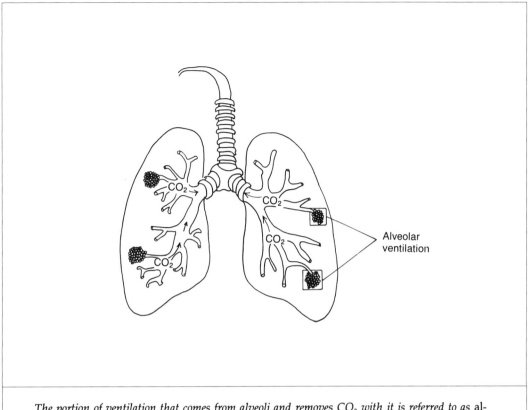

The portion of ventilation that comes from alveoli and removes CO_2 with it is referred to as alveolar ventilation (VA).

Once in the alveoli, CO_2 mixes with air and is removed from the lungs during _____.

ventilation

The portion of ventilation responsible for CO_2 removal is referred to as _____ _____.

alveolar ventilation

Note: The portion of ventilation that does not remove CO_2 or participate in gas exchange is called *dead space ventilation (VD)*. We can see that each tidal volume contains gas from two sources —the alveoli and the dead space:

$$V_T = V_A + V_D$$

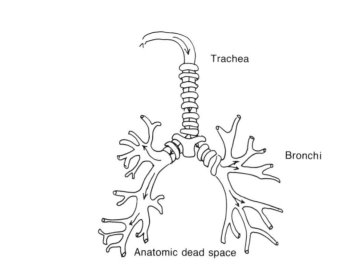

Trachea

Bronchi

Anatomic dead space

Ventilation of the upper and tracheobronchial airways, which contain no alveoli, is referred to as anatomic dead space *ventilation.*

Ventilation of the upper airway (e.g., nasopharynx, oropharynx, larynx) does not result in CO_2 elimination and is referred to as _____ _____ ventilation.

dead space

The tracheobronchial airways are part of the _____ dead space.

anatomic

Note: An estimate of the anatomic dead space can be made by multiplying the person's ideal body weight (in lb) by the factor of 1 cc per lb. For example, a 150 lb person would have approximately 150 cc of anatomic dead space.

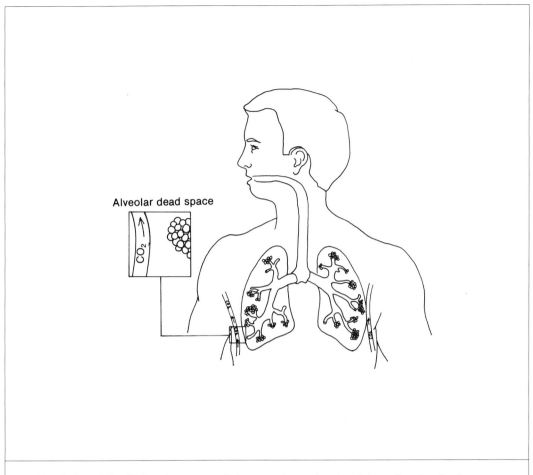

Alveolar dead space

CO_2

Ventilation of alveoli that does not result in gas exchange is referred to as alveolar dead space ventilation.

Note: Lung disease that results in ventilation of alveoli that do not have capillary perfusion will result in alveolar dead space. The classic example of this is a pulmonary embolus which results in the ventilation of unperfused alveoli.

Ventilation of alveoli that are not being _____ results in alveolar dead space.

perfused

Alveolar dead space occurs when ventilation of alveoli does not result in _____ _____ .

gas exchange

Dead space ventilation does not result in the removal of _____ from the lungs.

CO_2

Note: The term *physiologic dead space* is used to describe the total dead space (i.e., anatomic and alveolar).

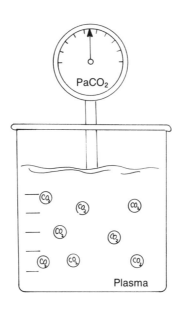

The arterial partial pressure of CO_2 (i.e., $PaCO_2$), reported in mmHg or torr, reflects the amount of CO_2 dissolved in plasma.

In ABG analysis, the CO_2 dissolved in arterial blood exerts a _____, which is called the $PaCO_2$.

pressure

The $PaCO_2$ is measured during _____ analysis.

ABG

Note: Recall that CO_2 is carried in the blood in several ways. The dissolved CO_2 exerts a pressure that is proportional to the total quantity carried in the blood. The majority of CO_2 combines with H_2O to form HCO_3^-, with Hb and other proteins carrying the remainder.

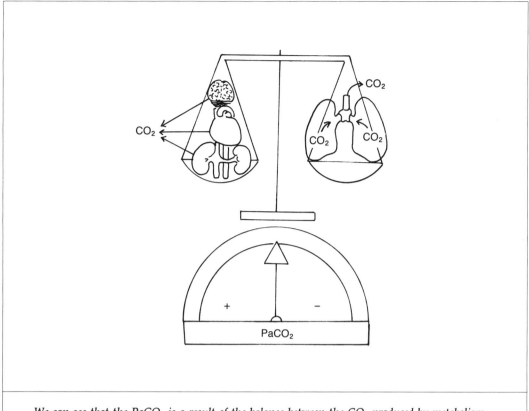

We can see that the $PaCO_2$ is a result of the balance between the CO_2 produced by metabolism and the amount removed by the lungs through alveolar ventilation.

CO_2 is _____ by metabolism and removed by alveolar ventilation.

produced

The $PaCO_2$ is the result of a _____ between the production and removal of the CO_2.

balance

Note: There is an inverse relationship between $PaCO_2$ and alveolar ventilation. As one increases, the other decreases and vice versa. Since the production of CO_2 by tissues is more or less constant, changes in $PaCO_2$ usually result from changes in alveolar ventilation.

The level of $PaCO_2$ is a direct measurement of _____ ventilation.

alveolar

The higher the alveolar ventilation, the _____ the $PaCO_2$.

lower

The lower the alveolar ventilation, the _____ the $PaCO_2$.

higher

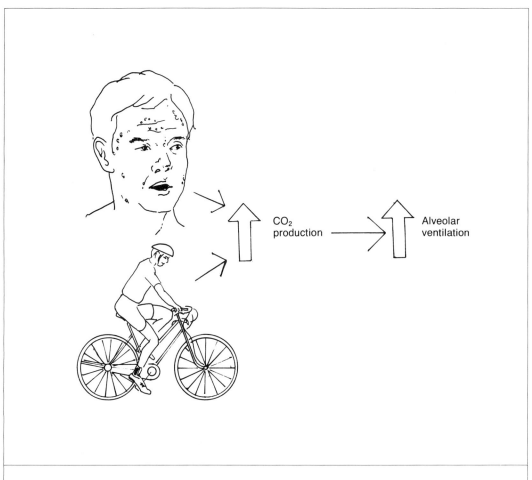

Any increase in metabolism (such as occurs with fever or exercise) will increase CO_2 production. In order to maintain the $PaCO_2$ at normal values, alveolar ventilation must increase accordingly.

With fever or exercise, there is an _____ in the production of CO_2.

increase

If production of CO_2 increases but removal remains the same, the $PaCO_2$ _____.

increases

In order to maintain a normal $PaCO_2$, as metabolism increases, alveolar _____ must also increase to remove excess CO_2.

ventilation

$PaCO_2$ is the result of the _____ between CO_2 production and its removal by alveolar ventilation.

balance

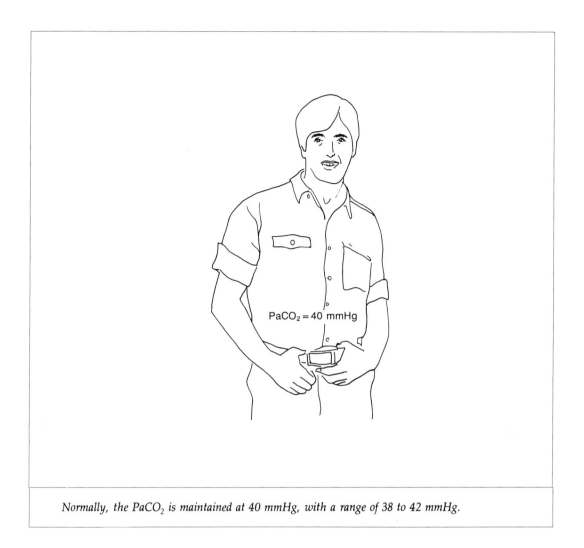

Normally, the PaCO$_2$ is maintained at 40 mmHg, with a range of 38 to 42 mmHg.

A normal PaCO$_2$ is _____.   *40 mmHg*

The balance between CO$_2$ production and elimination maintains
the PaCO$_2$ in the range of _____.   *38 to 42 mmHg*

Note: In spite of variations in daily activity, the PaCO$_2$ is normally maintained within a limited range.

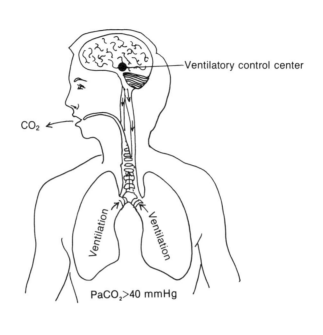

CO$_2$

Ventilatory control center

Ventilation

Ventilation

PaCO$_2$>40 mmHg

The medulla's ventilatory control center *regulates breathing to maintain the PaCO$_2$ in its normal range.*

Normally, the _____ _____ center will adjust breathing to keep pace with CO$_2$ production and to maintain PaCO$_2$ within a limited range.

ventilatory control

Breathing (or more specifically, alveolar ventilation) is regulated to keep the _____ within a limited range.

PaCO$_2$

The ventilatory control center is located in the _____.

medulla

Note: The ventilatory control center receives input from many sources (e.g., chemical sensors in the body that monitor O$_2$ and CO$_2$ levels as well as stretch receptors in the airways that monitor lung expansion). Conscious input from the higher brain can also control ventilation. The role of the ventilatory control center is to integrate all of these inputs and establish the breathing pattern.

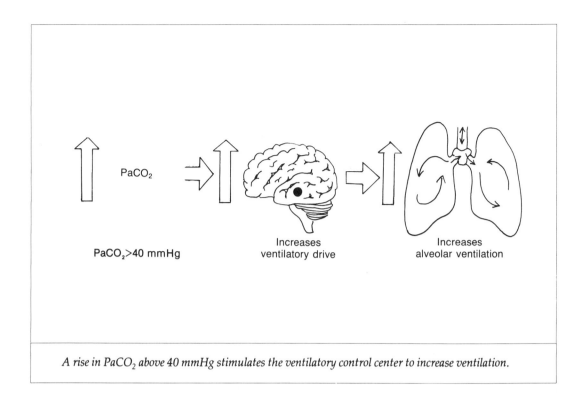

PaCO₂

PaCO$_2$>40 mmHg

Increases
ventilatory drive

Increases
alveolar ventilation

A rise in PaCO$_2$ above 40 mmHg stimulates the ventilatory control center to increase ventilation.

In response to a rise in PaCO$_2$ above 40 mmHg, the ventilatory control center is stimulated to _____ breathing.

increase

As alveolar ventilation increases, more CO$_2$ is removed and the PaCO$_2$ _____.

decreases

Note: A rise in PaCO$_2$ above 40 mmHg will usually stimulate the ventilatory control center to increase ventilation. The degree and effectiveness of this response will depend on many factors, including how well the respiratory muscles respond and the condition of the lungs. For example, because of severe lung dysfunction, a patient with advanced obstructive lung disease may not be able to increase alveolar ventilation in response to the signals from the ventilatory control center.

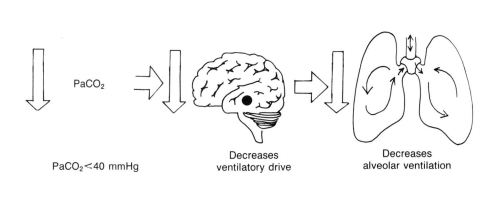

PaCO$_2$

PaCO$_2$<40 mmHg

Decreases
ventilatory drive

Decreases
alveolar ventilation

A decrease in PaCO$_2$ below 40 mmHg causes the ventilatory control center to decrease alveolar ventilation in an attempt to raise PaCO$_2$ back toward normal.

In response to a low PaCO$_2$, the ventilatory control center will attempt to _____ alveolar ventilation.

decrease

Note: Although a low PaCO$_2$ will decrease ventilatory drive, there are many other sources of input to the ventilatory control center. For example, a person with a low PaCO$_2$ who has pneumonia may continue to breathe excessively, leaving the PaCO$_2$ lower than normal.

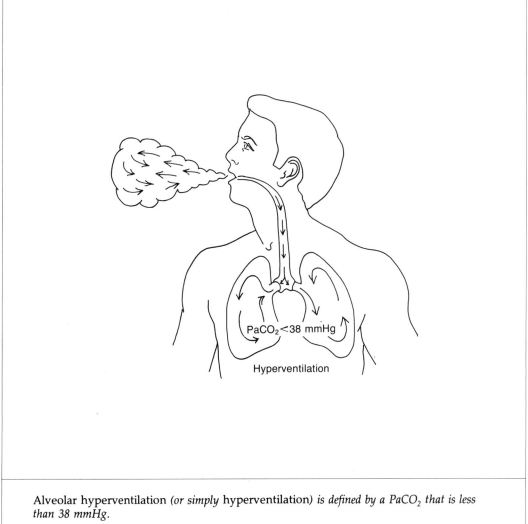

PaCO$_2$<38 mmHg

Hyperventilation

Alveolar hyperventilation *(or simply* hyperventilation*) is defined by a PaCO$_2$ that is less than 38 mmHg.*

A PaCO$_2$ less than _____ mmHg is defined as hyperventilation.

38

Hyperventilation is another way of saying that the PaCO$_2$ is _____.

low

Note: Rapid breathing (tachypnea) is often incorrectly referred to as hyperventilation. If rapid breathing is not causing a PaCO$_2$ below 38 mmHg, the person is *not* hyperventilating! In other words, hyperventilation can *only* be defined on the basis of the PaCO$_2$.

The diagnosis of hyperventilation must be based on the level of _____.

PaCO$_2$

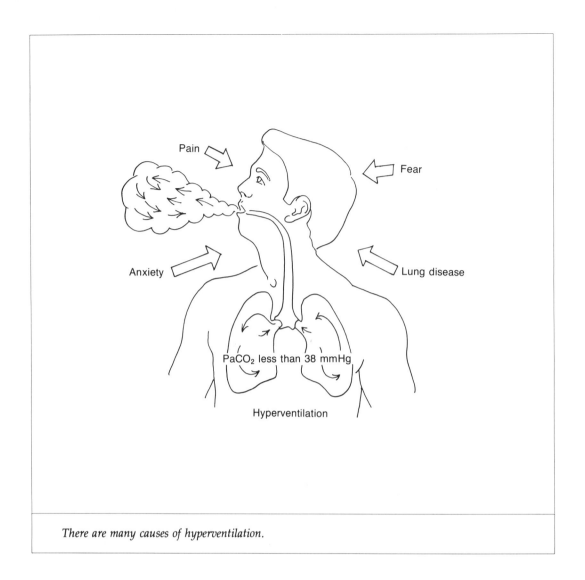

There are many causes of hyperventilation.

Anything that stimulates respiratory drive can lead to _____.

hyperventilation

Note: Pain, fear, and anxiety are some of the common causes of hyperventilation. Many lung diseases will cause an increase in breathing efforts and result in hyperventilation (unless the patient is too weak to respond to the stimulus or the lung disease is so severe that despite increased effort they are unable to increase alveolar ventilation).

Hyperventilation results whenever alveolar ventilation is excessive in relation to CO_2 _____.

production

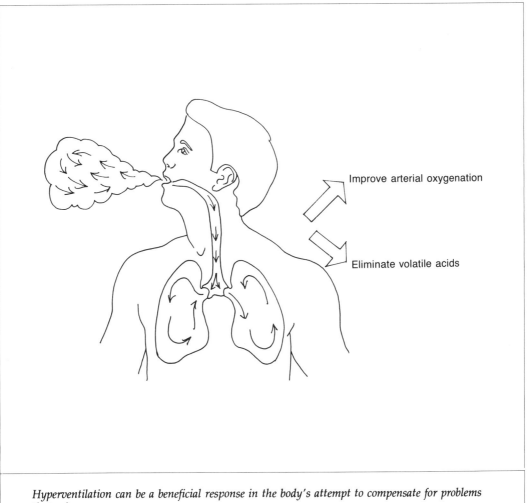

Improve arterial oxygenation

Eliminate volatile acids

Hyperventilation can be a beneficial response in the body's attempt to compensate for problems that arise.

A person will sometimes hyperventilate in an attempt to
_____ for a problem that has occurred.   *compensate*

Hyperventilation is sometimes a _____ response.   *beneficial*

Note: In response to a buildup of acid in the body, one may hyperventilate to lower the H_2CO_3 level and maintain acid-base balance (i.e., compensate for the acid buildup). In response to severe decreases in PaO_2, one may hyperventilate in an attempt to improve arterial oxygenation.

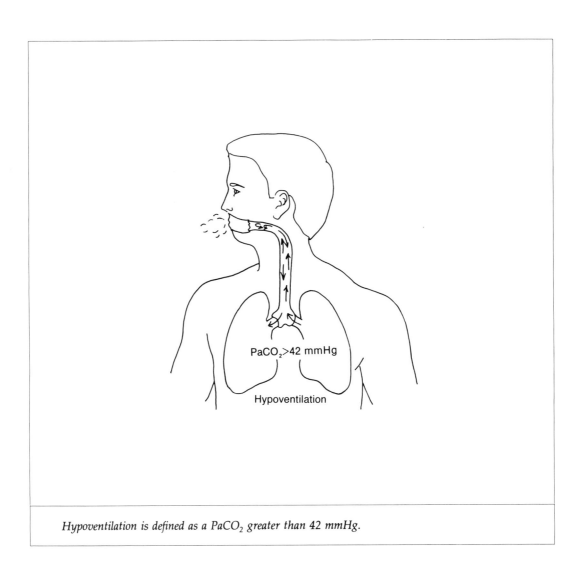

Hypoventilation is defined as a $PaCO_2$ greater than 42 mmHg.

Hypoventilation is associated with an _____ in $PaCO_2$.

increase

A $PaCO_2$ greater than _____ mmHg represents hypoventilation.

42

As alveolar ventilation decreases, less CO_2 is excreted by the lungs, causing the $PaCO_2$ to _____.

rise

Note: Neither hyperventilation nor hypoventilation can be diagnosed by simply looking at the patient or counting the respiratory rate. You must obtain an ABG for an accurate diagnosis.

$$V_T = 300 \text{ ml}$$

$$f = 24/\text{min}$$

$$PaCO_2 = 60 \text{ mmHg}$$

We can apply some of the concepts reviewed in the last few pages by assessing this patient's ventilatory status.

This patient's minute ventilation ($\dot{V}_E$) is _____ L per min.

7.2

Even though the patient is tachypneic (f = 24), the ventilatory status is best determined by measuring the _____.

PaCO$_2$

In assessing the patient's ventilatory status, we see that the $PaCO_2$ is 60 and conclude that the patient is _____.

hypoventilating

Note: Keep in mind that despite a rapid respiratory rate and relatively normal $\dot{V}_E$, this patient is hypoventilating. The conclusion to be drawn is that there must be a lot of wasted or dead space ventilation resulting in an overall decrease in alveolar ventilation, as indicated by the elevated $PaCO_2$.

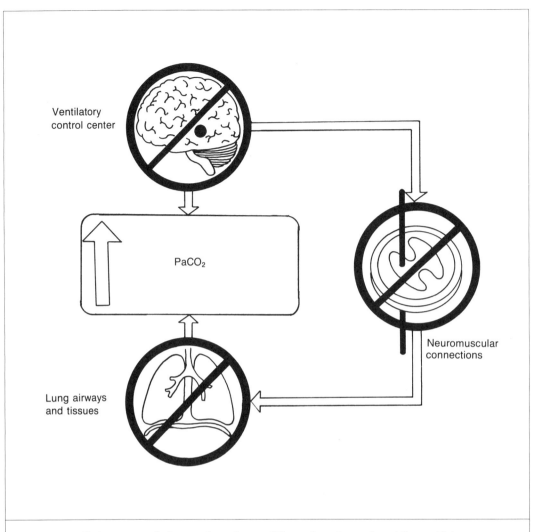

Hypoventilation can result from various abnormalities such as depression of the ventilatory control center (e.g., from narcotics), respiratory neuromuscular disorders (e.g., polio), or defects in the lung airways and tissues (e.g., advanced emphysema).

Depression of the ventilatory control center from _____ can cause hypoventilation.

narcotics

Respiratory muscle weakness from _____ disease can result in an increase in $PaCO_2$.

neuromuscular

Lung disease, particularly when in the advanced stages, can cause retention of _____.

CO_2

Note: *Hypercapnia* means a high $PaCO_2$ and is sometimes used in place of *hypoventilation*. Similarly, *hypocapnia* (a low $PaCO_2$) can be used in place of *hyperventilation*.

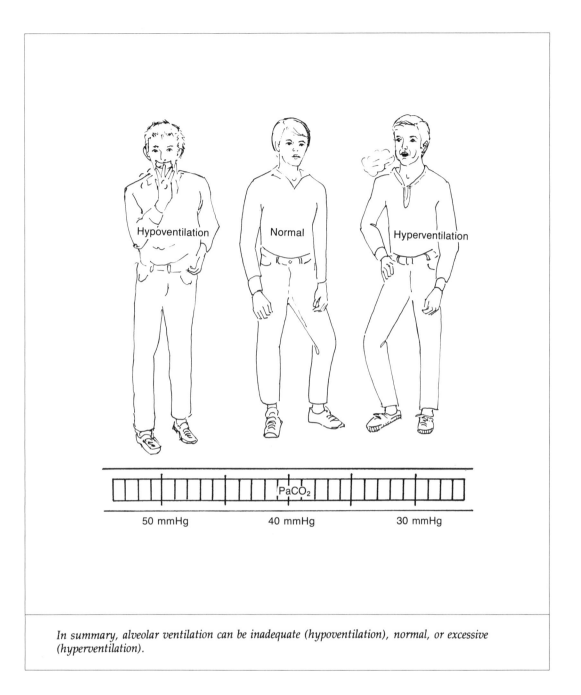

In summary, alveolar ventilation can be inadequate (hypoventilation), normal, or excessive (hyperventilation).

Excessive alveolar ventilation is called _____ and is defined by a $PaCO_2$ less than 38 mmHg.

hyperventilation

Normal alveolar ventilation is defined by a $PaCO_2$ in the range of _____ _____ .

38 to 42 mmHg

Inadequate alveolar ventilation is called _____ and is defined by a $PaCO_2$ greater than 42 mmHg.

hypoventilation

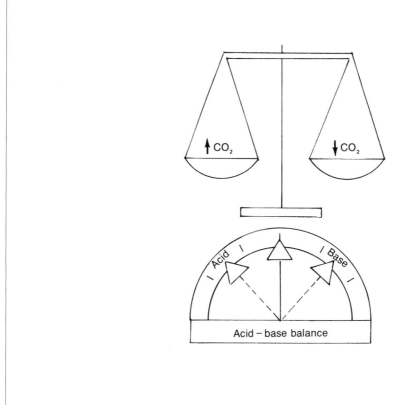

Since CO_2 combines with H_2O to form H_2CO_3, changes in the CO_2 level will affect the body's acid-base balance.

Increases in $PaCO_2$ cause an increase in the _____ _____ level of the blood.

acid

Changes in $PaCO_2$ will affect the acid-base _____ of the body.

balance

Note: A sudden buildup of CO_2 and hence acid in the blood will usually cause an acidemia, which is reflected in a decrease in the blood pH (<7.38). A fall in CO_2 (i.e., acid) will cause an alkalemia and this is reflected in an increase in pH (>7.42). (See Chap. 5).

Acute changes in PaCO$_2$ → Changes in pH

Acute changes in the PaCO$_2$ can have dramatic effects on the pH.

Changes that occur suddenly are referred to as _____ changes.

acute

Sudden changes in PaCO$_2$ can have dramatic effects on _____.

pH

When the PaCO$_2$ changes slowly, the body has more time to adjust and make compensatory changes. The effects are therefore usually not as _____ (or harmful)!

dramatic

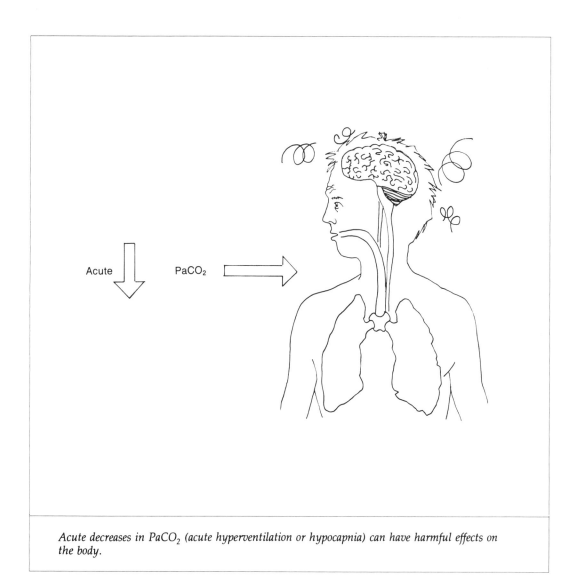

Acute PaCO$_2$

Acute decreases in PaCO$_2$ (acute hyperventilation or hypocapnia) can have harmful effects on the body.

Acute hyperventilation can have _____ effects.

harmful

With the loss of acid that occurs with a decrease in PaCO$_2$, the person may develop acute _____.

alkalemia

Note: Acute alkalemia may cause serious problems with nervous system conduction and result in electrical instability of the heart. A rapid fall in PaCO$_2$ can also cause vasoconstriction of cerebral vessels, resulting in decreased blood flow to the brain. This probably accounts for the dizziness that often accompanies hyperventilation.

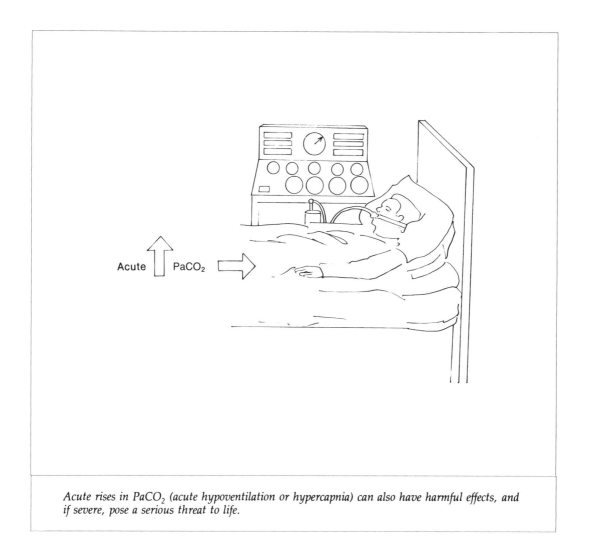

Acute rises in PaCO$_2$ (acute hypoventilation or hypercapnia) can also have harmful effects, and if severe, pose a serious threat to life.

A rapid increase in PaCO$_2$ will result in a sudden _____ in H$_2$CO$_3$.

increase

This buildup of acid can cause the _____ to become acidic.

blood

Note: Rapid accumulation of CO$_2$ may pose a threat to life for these reasons:

1. Sudden acidemia can affect heart and brain function.
2. Rapid rise in PaCO$_2$ can cause vasodilation, edema, and respiratory center depression.
3. Associated falls in PaO$_2$ can produce cardiac dysrhythmias and central nervous system damage.

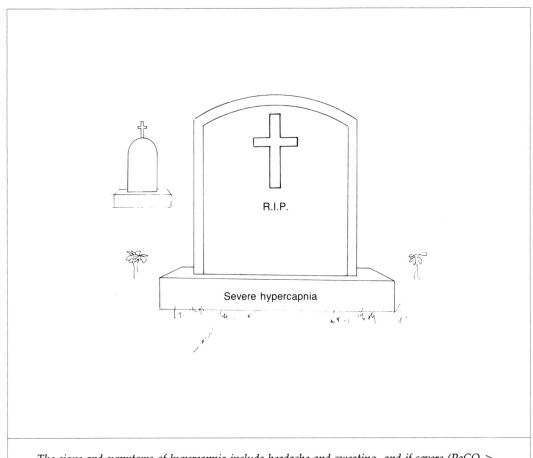

The signs and symptoms of hypercapnia include headache and sweating, and if severe (PaCO$_2$ > 80–90 mmHg), can result in lethargy and even coma or death.

Signs and symptoms of hypercapnia include headache and
_____.

sweating

Severe hypercapnia can cause lethargy and _____.

coma

Note: The signs and symptoms of hypercapnia are not very specific and can result from many other causes. An ABG is the only method of accurately diagnosing hypercapnia.

Bibliography

Braun, H. A., Cheney, F., and Loehnen, P. *Introduction to Respiratory Physiology* (2nd ed.). Boston: Little, Brown, 1980. Pp. 27–37.

Slonim, N. B., and Hamilton, L. H. *Respiratory Physiology* (5th ed.). St. Louis: Mosby, 1987. Pp. 53–64.

West, J. B. Causes of carbon dioxide retention in lung disease. *N. Engl. J. Med.* 284 : 22, 1971.

West, J. B. *Respiratory Physiology: The Essentials* (3rd ed.). Baltimore: Williams & Wilkins, 1985. Pp. 11–20.

4   Gas Exchange

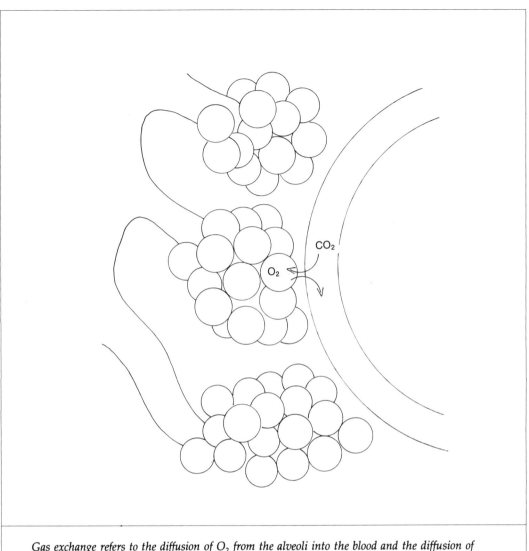

Gas exchange refers to the diffusion of O_2 from the alveoli into the blood and the diffusion of CO_2 from the blood into the alveoli.

_____ diffuses from alveoli into the blood.   *O_2*

CO_2 diffuses into the _____ from the blood.   *alveoli*

The diffusion of these gases into and out of the blood is referred
to as _____ _____.   *gas exchange*

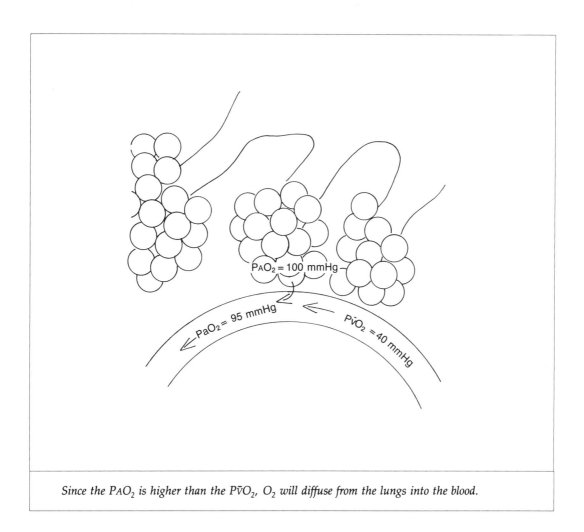

$P_{A}O_2 = 100$ mmHg

$PaO_2 = 95$ mmHg

$P\bar{v}O_2 = 40$ mmHg

Since the $P_{A}O_2$ is higher than the $P\bar{v}O_2$, O_2 will diffuse from the lungs into the blood.

Do you recall the normal values for alveolar and venous O_2 tensions?

When breathing room air, the $P_{A}O_2$ is normally _____ mmHg.

The normal $P\bar{v}O_2$ is _____ mmHg.

Since the $P_{A}O_2$ is greater than the $P\bar{v}O_2$, O_2 _____ into the blood.

100

40

diffuses

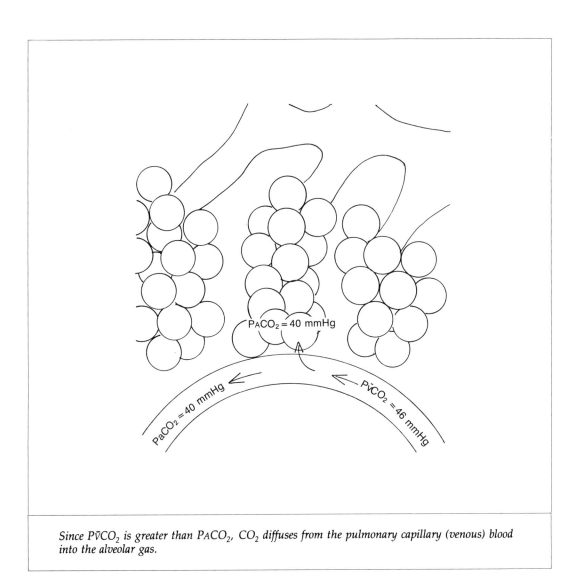

Since $P\bar{v}CO_2$ is greater than $PACO_2$, CO_2 diffuses from the pulmonary capillary (venous) blood into the alveolar gas.

The partial pressure of CO_2 in the pulmonary-capillary (venous)
blood is normally _____ mmHg.

46

The $PACO_2$ is normally _____ mmHg.

40

As a result of the partial pressure gradient, CO_2 diffuses from
the blood into the _____.

alveoli

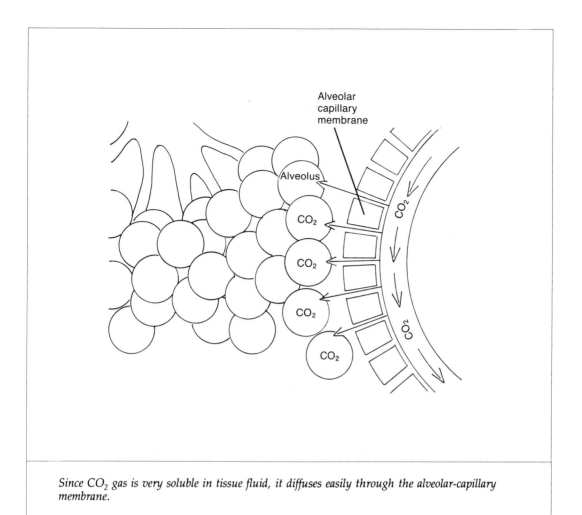

Since CO₂ gas is very soluble in tissue fluid, it diffuses easily through the alveolar-capillary membrane.

CO$_2$ gas is very _____ in tissue fluid.   *soluble*

Since CO$_2$ easily dissolves in the tissue fluid, it will readily
_____ through the alveolar-capillary membrane.   *diffuse*

Note: Because of its solubility in the tissue fluid, CO$_2$ is considered very diffusable through the alveolar-capillary membrane. As a result, the partial pressure of CO$_2$ gas in the blood leaving the lung has equilibrated with the partial pressure of CO$_2$ in the alveolar gas ($PaCO_2$ = $PACO_2$).

Arterial blood leaving alveoli has the same PCO$_2$ as the gas in
the _____.   *alveoli*

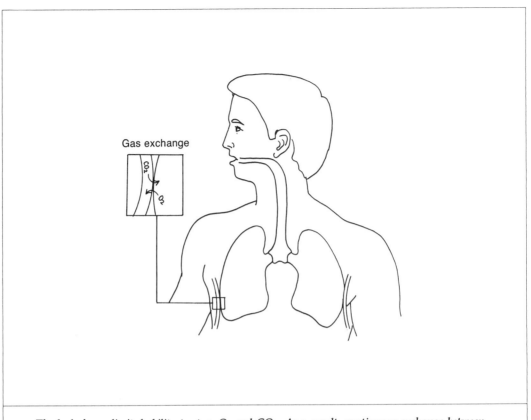

Gas exchange

The body has a limited ability to store O_2 and CO_2. As a result, continuous exchange between inspired air and pulmonary-capillary blood is necessary to maintain these gases at levels consistent with proper cellular function.

The body's ability to store O_2 and CO_2 is _____.

limited

In order to maintain a balance between the O_2 consumed and the CO_2 produced by cells, continuous _____ of these gases in the lungs is necessary.

exchange

Note: There are actually two sites of gas exchange. In the tissues, O_2 is consumed and CO_2 produced. This is referred to as *internal respiration*. In the lungs, O_2 is replenished and excess CO_2 eliminated. This is referred to as *external respiration*. When analyzing an ABG, we are provided with information that allows us to evaluate the gas exchange function of the lungs.

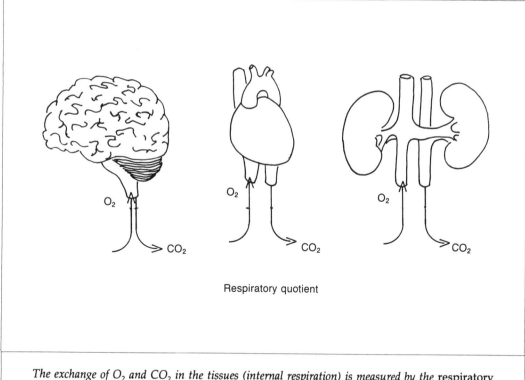

Respiratory quotient

The exchange of O_2 and CO_2 in the tissues (internal respiration) is measured by the respiratory quotient (RQ).

Gas exchange between the blood and tissues is known as
_____ respiration.

The exchange of gases at the tissue level is measured by the
_____.

Note: During internal respiration, O_2 is normally consumed at a rate of 250 cc per minute ($\dot{V}O_2$ = 250 ml/min) and CO_2 is produced at a rate of 200 cc per minute ($\dot{V}CO_2$ = 200 ml/min). The ratio of $\dot{V}CO_2/\dot{V}O_2$ or respiratory quotient (RQ) is normally 200/250 = 0.8. The RQ can vary from 0.7–1.0 depending on what fuel (i.e., glucose, protein, fats) is being metabolized for energy.

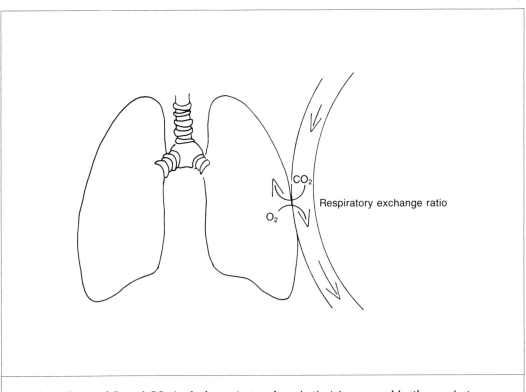

The exchange of O_2 and CO_2 in the lungs (external respiration) is measured by the respiratory exchange ratio (R).

The exchange of O_2 and CO_2 in the lungs is referred to as _____ respiration.

external

External respiration is measured by the respiratory exchange ratio and is expressed by the letter _____.

R

External respiration provides a measure of gas exchange in the _____.

lungs

Note: The rate at which CO_2 is eliminated by the lungs usually equals the rate at which it is produced by the tissues. Similarly, the rate at which O_2 is consumed by the tissues usually equals the amount of O_2 uptake by the lungs. A failure by the lungs to provide adequate gas exchange can result in either a buildup of CO_2 or a lack of O_2 in the blood.

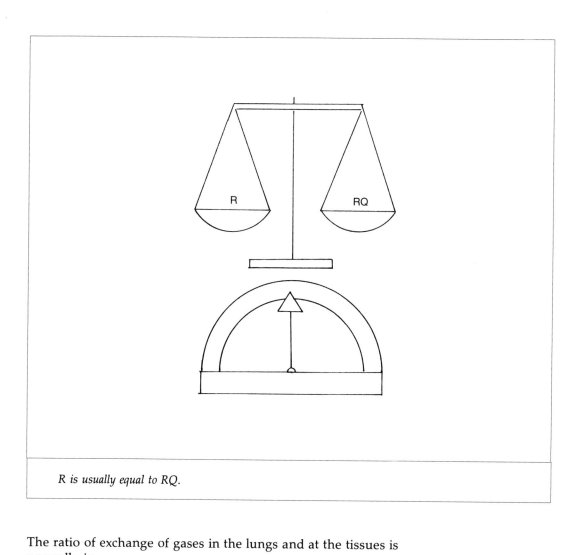

R is usually equal to RQ.

The ratio of exchange of gases in the lungs and at the tissues is normally in _____.

balance

Note: As long as the body maintains a balance (i.e., steady state or homeostasis), the consumption of O_2 and the production of CO_2 in the tissues (i.e., RQ) is matched by an equivalent exchange of gases in the lung (i.e., R).

Internal respiration in the tissues is usually balanced by _____ respiration in the lungs.

external

R and RQ are equal and have a numerical value of _____.

0.8

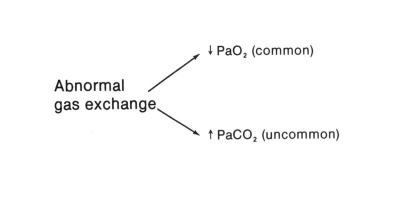

Abnormal gas exchange

↓ PaO_2 (common)

↑ $PaCO_2$ (uncommon)

Abnormal gas exchange will result in decreased transfer of O_2 into the blood (causing hypoxemia) or inadequate removal of CO_2 (causing hypercapnia) or both.

When gas exchange is abnormal, it interferes with _____ respiration.

external

Since CO_2 production is continuous, failure to eliminate it through the lungs will cause CO_2 to _____ in the blood.

accumulate

Since O_2 consumption is continuous, abnormal gas exchange will result in _____ oxygen levels in the blood.

decreased

By interfering with normal transfer of O_2 and CO_2 between the blood and lungs, impairment in gas exchange can cause _____ and possibly _____.

hypoxemia, hypercapnia

Gas exchange efficiency $\approx$ ABGs

The efficiency with which the lungs carry out gas exchange is reflected in the arterial blood gases.

Alveolar ventilation is responsible for elimination of _____ and replenishment of O_2 in the alveoli.

CO_2

Gas exchange across the alveolar-capillary membrane depends on _____ and matching of ventilation and perfusion.

diffusion

A breakdown in either of the above processes can result in abnormal _____ _____ in the lungs.

gas exchange

Abnormal gas exchange will be reflected in abnormalities in the _____.

ABGs

117

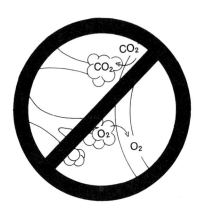

A decrease in the transfer of O_2 from the alveoli into the pulmonary-capillary blood is the most common type of gas exchange abnormality.

The most common type of gas exchange abnormality is a decreased transfer of _____ into the blood.

O_2

This decreased transfer causes _____ to develop.

hypoxemia

Note: Remember that hypoxemia is caused by one of four abnormalities? If needed, please review Chap. 2, p. 60.

The physiologic causes of hypoxemia are

1. _____
2. _____
3. _____
4. _____

V/Q mismatch
shunting
decreased PAO_2
diffusion defects

Note: A decrease in PAO_2 does not actually result from a gas exchange problem across the aveolar-capillary membrane but from problems with replenishing O_2 in the alveoli due to inadequate alveolar ventilation. V/Q mismatch, shunts, and diffusion defects cause insufficient transfer of O_2 across the alveolar-capillary membrane.

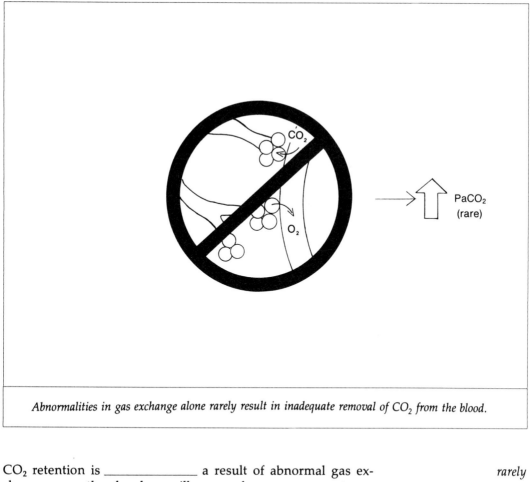

Abnormalities in gas exchange alone rarely result in inadequate removal of CO_2 from the blood.

CO_2 retention is _____ a result of abnormal gas exchange across the alveolar-capillary membrane.

rarely

Note: Because of the solubility of CO_2, it is able to move easily across the fluid-tissue layers from blood to alveolar gas. Retention of CO_2 is more likely to result from inadequate removal of the gas from the alveoli once it diffuses there (i.e., a decrease in alveolar ventilation).

CO_2 retention usually results from a decrease in _____ ventilation rather than from inadequate gas exchange.

alveolar

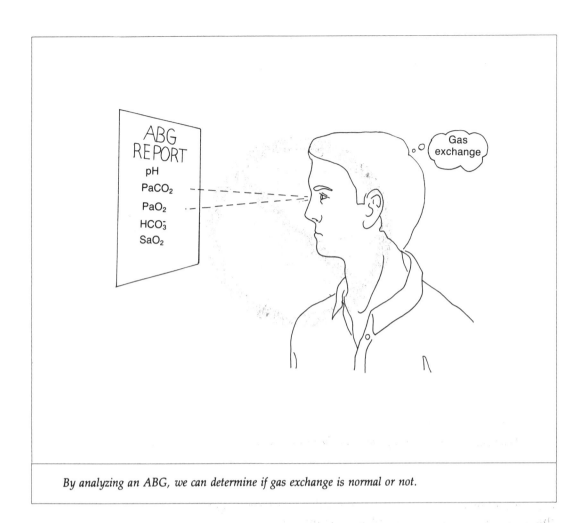

By analyzing an ABG, we can determine if gas exchange is normal or not.

ABG analysis will demonstrate whether gas exchange is
_____.

normal

The most common result of abnormal gas exchange is a fall in
the _____.

PaO_2

Note: Abnormalities in gas exchange indicate a problem with
the exchange of O_2 and CO_2 gas between alveoli and blood. A
decrease in PaO_2 is not the only indication of a gas exchange
problem. In some cases, the PaO_2 can be normal or even high
and the patient may still have a gas exchange problem. If the
PAO_2 is increased from breathing supplemental O_2 or from a decrease in $PACO_2$, the PaO_2 would be expected to be higher than
normal. In these cases, evaluation of the alveolar-arterial O_2 tension gradient (A-aDO_2) will allow us to detect the abnormality in
gas exchange.

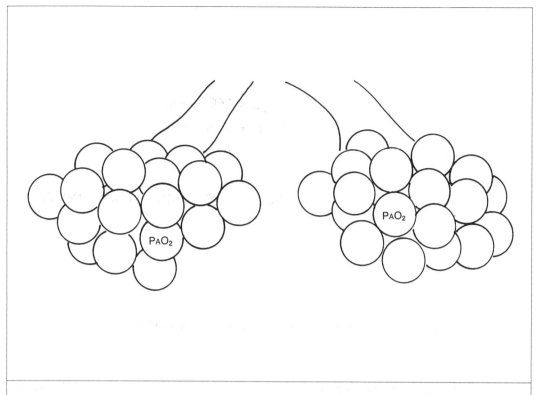

To calculate the A-aDO$_2$, we must first know the level of PO$_2$ in the average alveolus (i.e., the PAO$_2$).

Note: The PAO$_2$ in the average alveolus is calculated by using the *alveolar air equation:*

$$PAO_2 = [FIO_2 \times (P_{atm} - PH_2O)] - PaCO_2/R$$

Review the definitions of the above symbols:

1. FIO$_2$ is the fraction of inspired O$_2$ (room air FIO$_2$ is 0.21).
2. P$_{atm}$ is atmospheric pressure and PH$_2$O refers to water vapor pressure. In the lung, these are usually 760 mmHg and 47 mmHg, respectively.
3. The PaCO$_2$, or pressure of CO$_2$ in the arterial blood, is usually 40 mmHg.
4. R is assumed to be 0.8.

The above values are usually used unless specific measurements indicate different values should be used.

For room air at sea level, the PAO$_2$ is calculated as follows:

$$[0.21 \times (760 - 47)] - 40/0.8 \approx 100 \text{ mmHg}$$

Assuming: $P_{atm} = 760$ mmHg

$PH_2O = 47$ mmHg

$R = 0.8$

Then:

$$PAO_2 = (713 \times FIO_2) - (1.25 \times PaCO_2)$$

If the typical assumptions are made, the alveolar air equation can be simplified.

P_{atm} is usually assumed to be equal to _____.   *760 mmHg*

PH_2O is assumed to be _____.   *47 mmHg*

R is assumed to be equal to _____.   *0.8*

Note: Using these typical assumptions, the equation can be simplified as follows:

Since $(P_{atm} - PH_2O) = (760 - 47) = 713$, and

$PaCO_2/0.8 = PaCO_2 \times 1.25$, the formula can be written as follows:

$$PAO_2 = (713 \times FIO_2) - (1.25 \times PaCO_2)$$

$$A\text{-}aDO_2 = PAO_2 - PaO_2$$

$$A\text{-}aDO_2 = [FIO_2\,(713) - PaCO_2\,(1.25)] - PaO_2$$

For room air (i.e., $FIO_2 = 0.21$)

$$A\text{-}aDO_2 = [150 - (1.25 \times PaCO_2)] - PaO_2$$

Gas exchange is evaluated by the $A\text{-}aDO_2$, which can be quickly and easily calculated.

Note: Utilizing the alveolar air equation, the formula for calculating the $A\text{-}aDO_2$ at any FIO_2 can be generalized as follows:

$$A\text{-}aDO_2 = PAO_2 - PaO_2$$
$$= [(713 \times FIO_2) - (1.25 \times PaCO_2)] - PaO_2$$

One method of estimating the $A\text{-}aDO_2$ on room air is as follows:

$$A\text{-}aDO_2 = [150 - (1.25 \times PaCO_2) - PaO_2$$

To calculate the $A\text{-}aDO_2$ of a patient breathing room air, simply subtract the value of PaO_2 and 1.25 times the value of $PaCO_2$ from 150. The 150 represents the estimated value of inspired oxygen on room air [i.e., $(P_{atm} - P_{H_2O})\,FIO_2$ or $(760 - 47) \times 0.21$].

What is the $A\text{-}aDO_2$ of a person who is breathing room air and has a normal $PaCO_2$? _____ mmHg   *10*

Using the simplified formula, here is the calculation for review:

$$A\text{-}aDO_2 = [150 - (1.25 \times 40)] - 90$$
$$= 100 - 90$$
$$\approx 10\ mmHg$$

Note: The maximal normal $A\text{-}aDO_2$ is 10 to 12 mmHg.

$$pH = 7.40$$
$$PaO_2 = 88 \text{ mmHg}$$
$$PaCO_2 = 40 \text{ mmHg}$$

Mrs. Clark is breathing a 40 percent O_2 mixture. What is the A-aDO_2 in this situation?

The A-aDO_2 is _____ mmHg.   147.2

If you need to review, the calculation is as follows:

$$
\begin{aligned}
\text{A-a}DO_2 &= [FIO_2 (713) - PaCO_2 (1.25)] - PaO_2 \\
&= [0.40 (713) - 40 (1.25)] - 88 \\
&= [285.2 - 50] - 88 \\
&= 147.2
\end{aligned}
$$

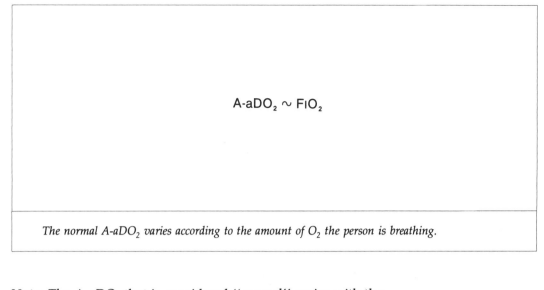

$$A\text{-aDO}_2 \sim F_{IO_2}$$

The normal A-aDO₂ varies according to the amount of O₂ the person is breathing.

Note: The $A\text{-aDO}_2$ that is considered "normal" varies with the F_{IO_2} the patient is breathing. The higher the O_2 percentage, the higher the anticipated $A\text{-aDO}_2$. There are complex physiologic reasons for this but, simply, one should expect an increased gradient as one breathes higher concentrations of O_2. The expected gradient increases proportionally from 5 to 10 mmHg when breathing room air ($F_{IO_2} = 0.21$) to approximately 120 mmHg when breathing 100 percent O_2 ($F_{IO_2} = 1.0$).

The normal $A\text{-aDO}_2$ _____ according to the O_2 percentage inspired.

varies

$A\text{-aDO}_2$ will _____ as the F_{IO_2} is increased.

increase

Note: The increased $A\text{-aDO}_2$ seen with breathing higher F_{IO_2}s does *not* represent a lung problem unless the increased gradient is greater than that anticipated as discussed above.

$$pH = 7.52$$

$$PaCO_2 = 32 \text{ mmHg}$$

$$PaO_2 = 600 \text{ mmHg}$$

Mr. Jones is breathing 100 percent oxygen with the above ABG results.

Note: Use R = 1.0. (This is usually assumed for patients who are on 100 percent O_2.)

Calculate the A-aDO_2: _____   *81 mmHg*

Would this be considered a normal PaO_2 for a person breathing this FIO_2? _____   *yes*

Note: When breathing 100 percent O_2, it is acceptable for the maximum A-aDO_2 to be 120 mmHg or less. In this case, it was only 81 mmHg, a value well within acceptable limits.

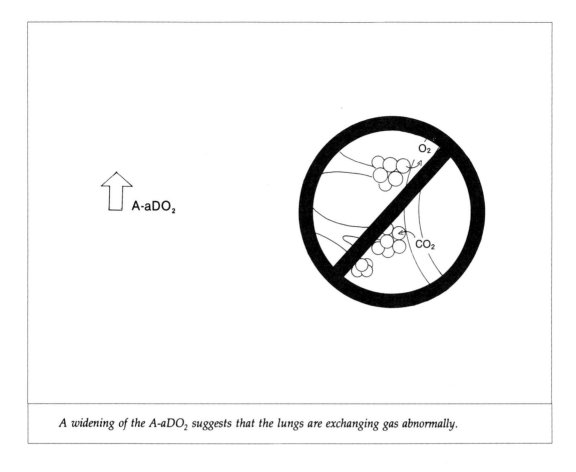

A widening of the $A\text{-}aDO_2$ suggests that the lungs are exchanging gas abnormally.

As gas exchange in the lung becomes abnormal, the _____ increases.

$A\text{-}aDO_2$

An increase in the $A\text{-}aDO_2$ is indicative of _____ disease.

lung

Note: As a general rule, the higher the $A\text{-}aDO_2$ gradient (above expected values), the greater the gas-exchange problem and the greater the severity of the lung disease.

Patient A	Patient B
pH $= 7.32$	pH $= 7.33$
$PaCO_2 = 57\,mmHg$	$PaCO_2 = 56\,mmHg$
$PaO_2 = 72\,mmHg$	$PaO_2 = 61\,mmHg$

Calculation of the A-aDO$_2$ can provide important clues to the presence of underlying lung disease.

In the above situation, two patients are diagnosed as having narcotic overdose.

Which patient has a gas-exchange problem? _____   *B*

Both patients have ABG evidence of _____ and   *hypoxemia*
_____, but only patient B is actually having difficulty   *hypercapnia*
with gas exchange across the alveolar-capillary membrane, as
evidenced by the increased _____ gradient.   *A-aDO$_2$*

Note: If ABGs reveal an increase in CO_2 but a normal A-aDO$_2$, the CO_2 retention is probably due to inadequate alveolar ventilation rather than a gas-exchange abnormality. If subsequent ABGs show widening of the A-aDO$_2$, this indicates superimposed lung disease in addition to hypoventilation. (Patient B was diagnosed as having aspiration pneumonia in addition to the drug overdose.)

Patient A is on a 40 percent Venturi O_2 mask and has the following ABGs:

$$pH = 7.34$$

$$PaCO_2 = 44 \text{ mmHg}$$

$$PaO_2 = 92 \text{ mmHg}$$

Patient B is on an aerosol mask on 30 percent O_2 and has the following ABGs (The $P_{atm} = 742$ mmHg in this situation):

$$pH = 7.41$$

$$PaCO_2 = 38 \text{ mmHg}$$

$$PaO_2 = 146 \text{ mmHg}$$

Calculate the A-aDO_2 in the above situations and compare the degree of severity of these patients' lung problems.

What is the A-aDO$_2$ in patient A? _____   *138.2 mmHg*

What is the A-aDO$_2$ in patient B? _____   *15 mmHg*

Which patient has the greater gas-exchange problem? _____   *A*

Which patient has the more severe lung disease? _____   *A*

Note: Of course the patient with the largest A-aDO$_2$ is assumed to have more severe lung disease.

$$PaO_2 \approx (713 \times FiO_2) - (1.25 \times PaCO_2)$$

By utilizing the alveolar air equation we can also check to see if the PaO_2 is consistent with the FiO_2 and the $PaCO_2$.

Note: The above is a simplified form of the alveolar air equation. The PaO_2 can, at best, be approximately equal to or slightly less than the alveolar PO_2. In the presence of an increased $A\text{-}aDO_2$, the PaO_2 may be less than the PaO_2. If the PaO_2 (as measured by blood gas analysis) is *greater* than the PaO_2 (as calculated from the above equation), then there is most likely an error in one of three places:

1. The patient is actually on a *higher* FiO_2 than reported.
2. There has been a laboratory error in measurement.
3. There has been a miscommunication between personnel in the laboratory and the person receiving the data.

If the PaO_2 reported in an ABG report is lower than the PaO_2, this indicates an _____ $A\text{-}aDO_2$.

increased

If the PaO_2 is greater than the PaO_2, an _____ has been made.

error

Bibliography

Dantzker, D. Physiology and pathophysiology of pulmonary gas exchange. *Hosp. Pract.*, January, 1986.

Moser, K. Oxygen and carbon dioxide transfer. *Respiratory Care*, 20 : 5, 1975.

West, J. B. New advances in pulmonary gas exchange. *Anesth. Analg.* 54 : 4, 1975.

West, J. B. *Respiratory Physiology: The Essentials* (3rd ed.). Baltimore Williams & Wilkins, 1985. Pp. 49–66.

West, J. B. Ventilation perfusion relationships. *Am. Rev. Respir. Dis.* 116 : 919, 1977.

5   *Acid-Base Balance*

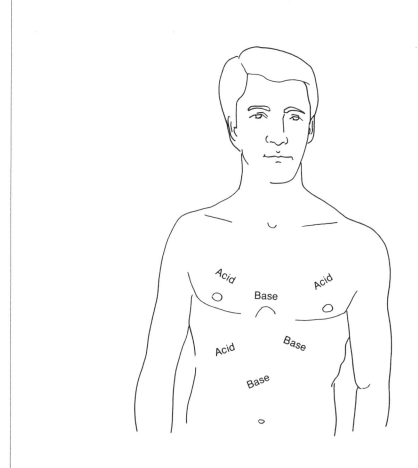

In addition to other substances, body fluids contain a mixture of chemicals known as acids and bases.

Body fluids contain a number of acids and _____.   *bases*

Note: Normally, the amounts of acids and bases in our body fluids are in balance and their relative proportions are maintained constant.

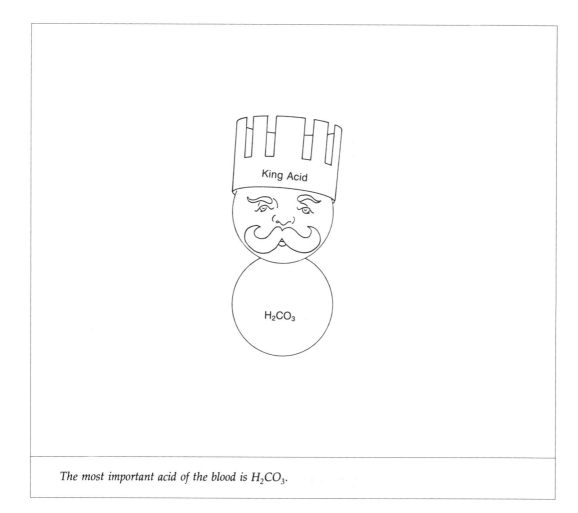

The most important acid of the blood is H_2CO_3.

Note: Acids are substances that can release H^+ into a solution. The greater the tendency to release H^+, the more acidic the substance (i.e., the stronger the acid). If H^+ is present in a substance but is not released into solution, the acidity of the solution is not affected.

It is the concentration of free H^+ that gives a solution its

_____.   *acidity*

H_2CO_3 is the most important _____ in the blood.   *acid*

H_2CO_3 can release _____ into solution and is therefore   *H^+*
an acid.

A strong acid can release more H^+ into solution than a

_____ acid.   *weak*

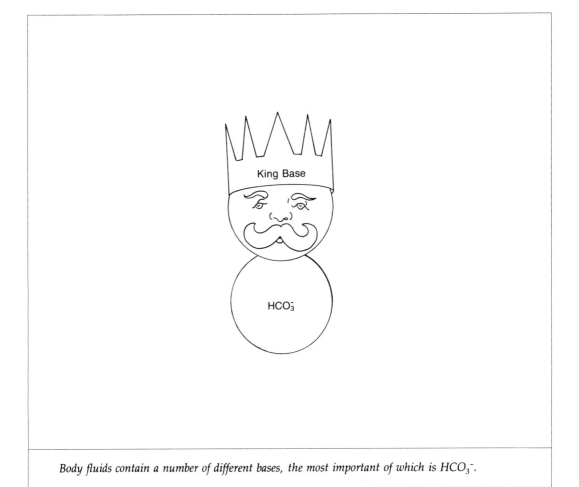

Body fluids contain a number of different bases, the most important of which is HCO_3^-.

Note: Bases are substances that can "accept," or chemically combine with, H^+. These substances reduce the number of free H^+ in the solution.

_____ is the most important base in the body.

_____ is the chemical symbol for bicarbonate.

Bicarbonate

HCO_3^-

Note: The amount of HCO_3^- in the blood is expressed in units of mEq/L. The normal concentration is 22 to 26 mEq/L. This is often expressed as $[HCO_3^-]$ = 22–26 mEq/L. The brackets indicate that we are dealing with the *concentration* of the substance.

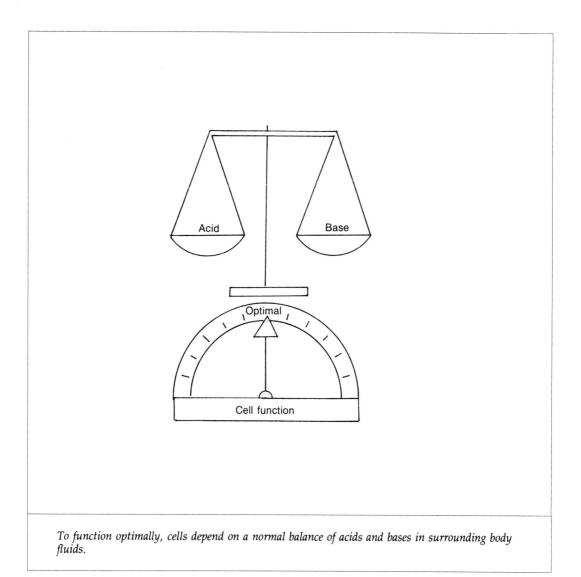

To function optimally, cells depend on a normal balance of acids and bases in surrounding body fluids.

Abnormally low or high concentrations of acids or bases in body fluids can interefere with cellular _____.

function

When the amounts of acid and base are normal, they are said to be in _____.

balance

Acid-base _____ can cause malfunction of cells, with potentially harmful consequences.

imbalances

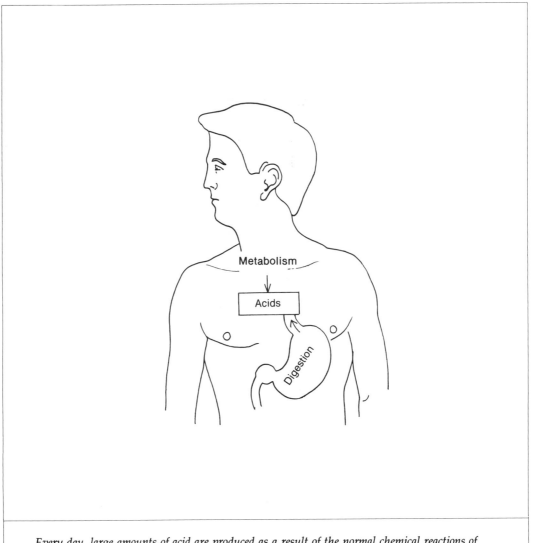

Every day, large amounts of acid are produced as a result of the normal chemical reactions of metabolism and digestion.

Large amounts of acid are produced each day from the processes of metabolism and _____.

digestion

Note: Acids produced by metabolism can be volatile or nonvolatile (fixed). Volatile acids are acids that can be removed from the body as a gas. H_2CO_3 is the primary volatile acid of body fluids and can be eliminated as CO_2 gas. Nonvolatile acids are also produced in small amounts by metabolism and are removed from the body via the kidney.

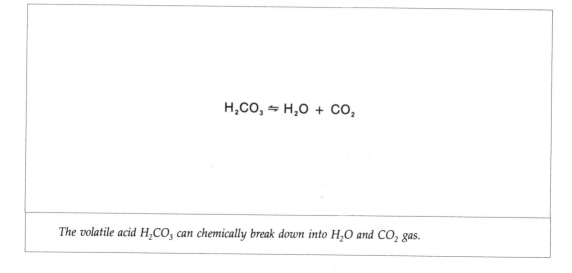

$$H_2CO_3 \rightleftharpoons H_2O + CO_2$$

The volatile acid H_2CO_3 can chemically break down into H_2O and CO_2 gas.

Note: H_2CO_3 is not easy to measure directly, but we can take advantage of the fact that the $[H_2CO_3]$ is directly proportional to the amount of CO_2 dissolved in the blood. This dissolved CO_2 may be expressed by the solubility constant (K) and the PCO_2 (i.e., $[H_2CO_3] \approx$ dissolved $CO_2 = PCO_2 \times K$). By virtue of this relationship, the $PaCO_2$ provides a measure of the amount of H_2CO_3 in the arterial blood.

The $PaCO_2$ can provide us with a measure of the _____ concentration of the arterial blood.

H_2CO_3

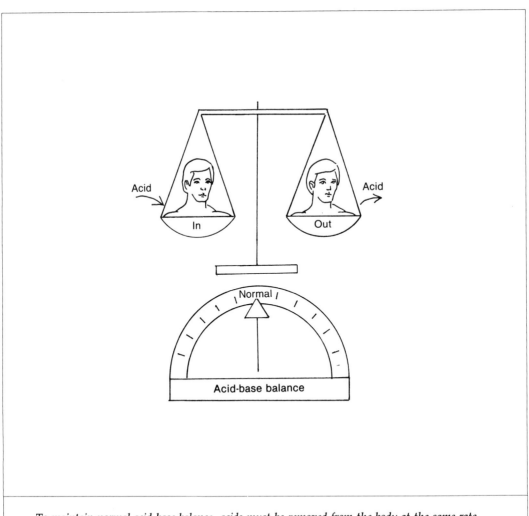

To maintain normal acid-base balance, acids must be removed from the body at the same rate that they are produced.

The body must remove excess acid in order to maintain acid-base
_____.

balance

Both volatile and _____ acids are produced and excreted by the body.

nonvolatile

If removal of acid does not keep pace with production, the result will be an acid-base _____.

imbalance

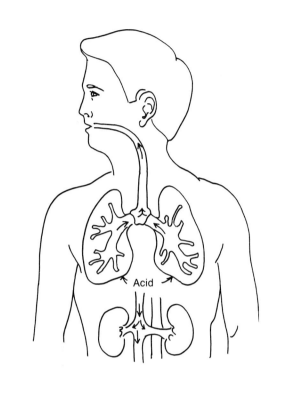

Acid

Acids produced in tissues throughout the body are ultimately eliminated at two sites—the lungs and the kidneys.

Although acids are produced in tissues throughout the body, they are eliminated at primarily _____ sites.

two

Most of the daily acid load is removed either by the lungs or by the _____.

kidneys

The lungs and kidneys remove acids and play an important role in maintaining _____ balance.

acid-base

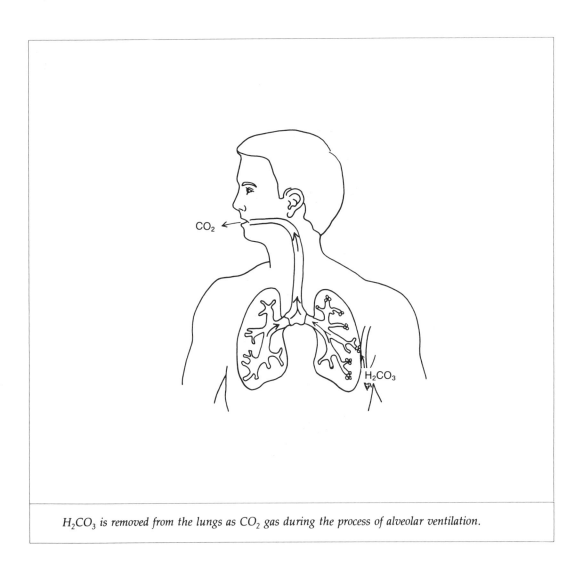

H_2CO_3 is removed from the lungs as CO_2 gas during the process of alveolar ventilation.

H_2CO_3 is a volatile acid that is eliminated from the body as
_____ gas.   *CO_2*

To maintain acid-base _____, H_2CO_3 is removed by   *balance*
the lungs as CO_2 gas.

The lungs help regulate acid-base balance by changes in alveolar
_____.   *ventilation*

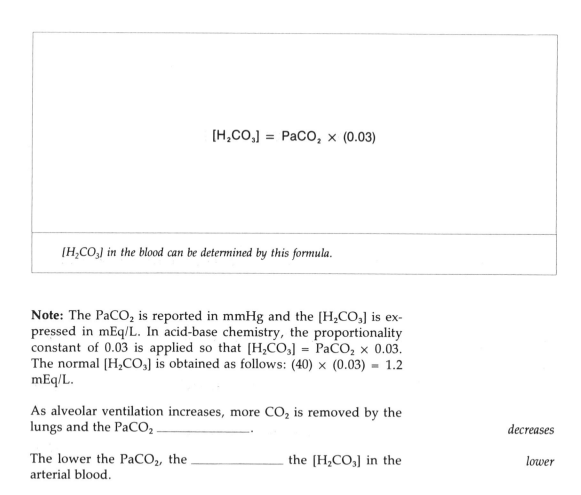

$$[H_2CO_3] = PaCO_2 \times (0.03)$$

[H₂CO₃] in the blood can be determined by this formula.

Note: The $PaCO_2$ is reported in mmHg and the $[H_2CO_3]$ is expressed in mEq/L. In acid-base chemistry, the proportionality constant of 0.03 is applied so that $[H_2CO_3] = PaCO_2 \times 0.03$. The normal $[H_2CO_3]$ is obtained as follows: $(40) \times (0.03) = 1.2$ mEq/L.

As alveolar ventilation increases, more CO_2 is removed by the lungs and the $PaCO_2$ _____.

decreases

The lower the $PaCO_2$, the _____ the $[H_2CO_3]$ in the arterial blood.

lower

$$\triangle \text{PaCO}_2 \ = \ \triangle \text{H}_2\text{CO}_3 \ = \ \triangle \text{pH}$$

Changes in alveolar ventilation (i.e., PaCO$_2$) that alter the [H$_2$CO$_3$] will have marked effects on acid-base balance.

The _____ is regulated by changes in alveolar ventilation.

PaCO$_2$

Changes in PaCO$_2$ will affect the _____ in the arterial blood.

[H$_2$CO$_3$]

[H$_2$CO$_3$] is a key component in regulating the body's acid-base _____.

balance

$$PaCO_2 \approx H_2CO_3 = \text{Respiratory component}$$

Since the PaCO$_2$ reflects the [H$_2$CO$_3$], it is known as the respiratory *component of acid-base balance.*

H$_2$CO$_3$ is a volatile _____ that is removed by the lungs as CO$_2$ gas.

acid

The PaCO$_2$ provides a _____ of the [H$_2$CO$_3$].

measure

The PaCO$_2$ is known as the _____ component of acid-base balance.

respiratory

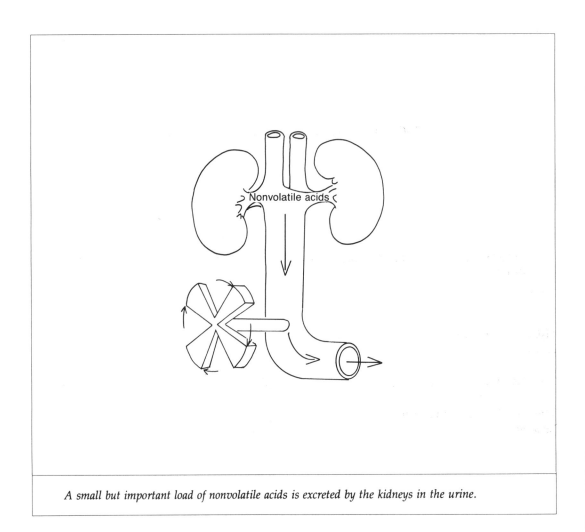

A small but important load of nonvolatile acids is excreted by the kidneys in the urine.

Nonvolatile acids produced by cellular metabolism are those acids that cannot be removed from the body as a _____.

gas

Nonvolatile acids are excreted by the _____ in the urine.

kidneys

Note: The major sources of nonvolatile acids are dietary intake, keto acids, and lactic acid. The kidneys excrete 50 to 100 mEq of nonvolatile acids per day. In contrast, the lungs excrete approximately 13,000 mEq of H_2CO_3 each day (in the form of CO_2 gas). Although kidney failure can cause accumulation of acid, it should be obvious why respiratory failure can produce a life-threatening acid accumulation much more rapidly.

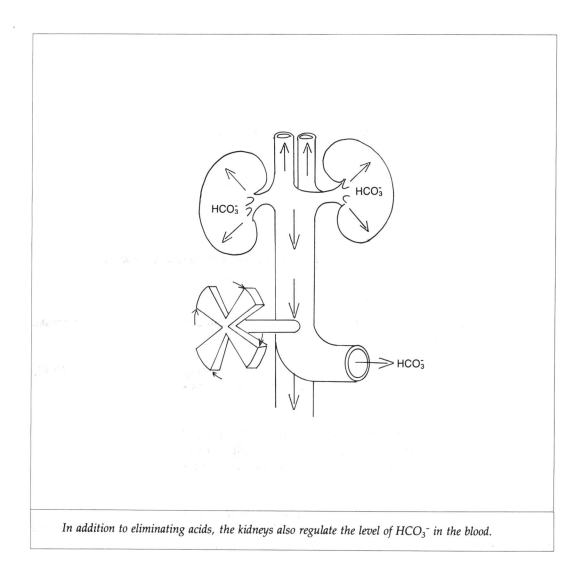

In addition to eliminating acids, the kidneys also regulate the level of HCO_3^- in the blood.

The level of HCO_3^- in the blood is regulated by the _____.

kidneys

Through their regulation of HCO_3^-, the kidneys play a vital role in maintaining acid-base _____.

balance

Note: The kidneys regulate the $[HCO_3^-]$ by increasing or decreasing the rate of resorption of HCO_3^- in the renal tubule.

$$[HCO_3^-] \approx \text{Metabolic component}$$

The level of HCO$_3^-$ can be used to reflect the metabolic component of acid-base balance.

The level of blood HCO$_3^-$ reflects the _____ component of acid-base balance.

metabolic

Through their regulation of _____, the kidneys play an important role in regulating the metabolic component of acid-base balance.

HCO$_3^-$

Note: Nonkidney-related problems can alter the level of HCO$_3^-$ and cause a metabolic acid-base imbalance. For example, electrolyte disturbances such as chloride depletion can result in retention of HCO$_3^-$.

Metabolic imbalances can result from nonkidney problems such as an _____ disturbance. (See pp. 243–245 for a brief review of electrolyte disturbances and acid-base imbalance.)

electrolyte

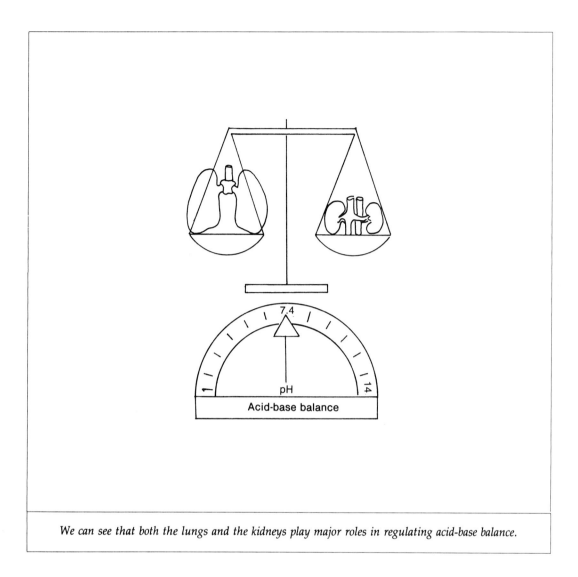

We can see that both the lungs and the kidneys play major roles in regulating acid-base balance.

The lungs regulate the level of _____ in the blood.

H_2CO_3

The $PaCO_2$, and hence $[H_2CO_3]$, is known as the _____ component of acid-base balance.

respiratory

The kidneys regulate the level of _____ in the blood.

HCO_3^-

The $[HCO_3^-]$ reflects the _____ component of acid-base balance.

metabolic

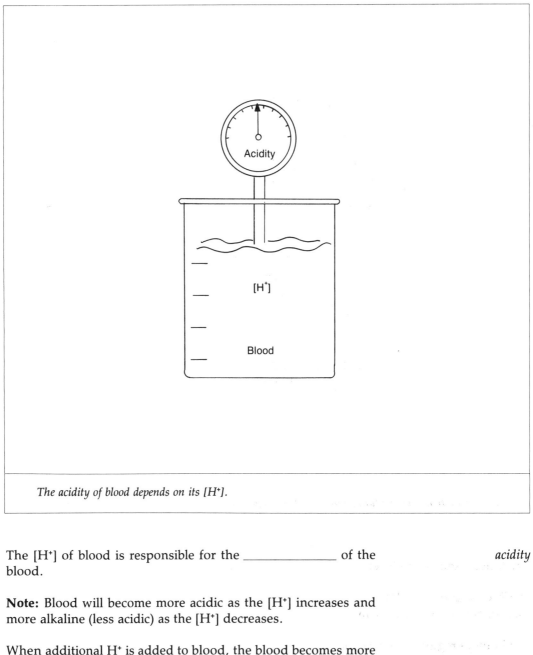

The acidity of blood depends on its [H⁺].

The [H⁺] of blood is responsible for the _____ of the blood.

acidity

Note: Blood will become more acidic as the [H⁺] increases and more alkaline (less acidic) as the [H⁺] decreases.

When additional H⁺ is added to blood, the blood becomes more _____.

acidic

When H⁺ is removed from blood, the blood becomes less acidic, or more _____.

alkaline

The acidity or alkalinity of blood is determined by the _____.

[H⁺]

$$pH \approx [H^+]$$

To express the [H⁺] (or acidity) of blood, we can use pH.

Note: The term *pH* is used to represent the concentration of free H⁺ in a solution. The pH of a solution is inversely proportional to the concentration of free H⁺ (i.e., as [H⁺] increases, the pH decreases and vice versa). Mathematically, pH = log 1/[H⁺]. To express [H⁺], however, requires very awkward numbers that do not help clarify the concepts of acidity and alkalinity. Alternatively, we can emphasize the importance of relative changes in [H⁺] by using pH and thereby avoid the confusion of trying to express the actual numbers of free H⁺ in a solution.

The [H⁺] of blood can be expressed by the _____.

     pH

As the pH increases, the [H⁺] in the solution _____.

     decreases

As the pH decreases, the _____ in the solution increases.

     [H⁺]

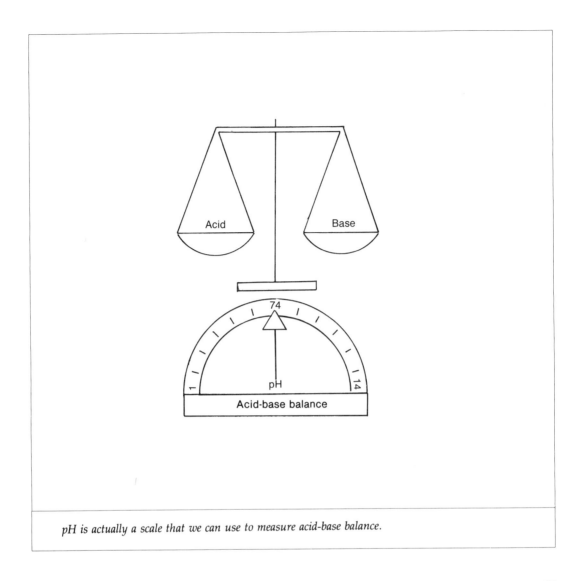

pH is actually a scale that we can use to measure acid-base balance.

To measure acid-base balance, we can use the _____.

pH

Note: The pH scale ranges from 1 to 14. A pH of 1 is the most acidic value, while a pH of 14 represents the most alkaline value. A pH of 7 is considered neutral.

A pH greater than 7 is considered _____, while a pH less than 7 is considered _____.

alkalotic
acidotic

Note: From a pure chemistry point of view, a pH of greater than 7 represents an alkaline pH. However, since arterial blood pH is normally 7.38 to 7.42, only pH greater than 7.42 is considered alkaline for blood. For the same reason, a pH less than 7.38 is referred to as an acidic pH.

Approximate relationship between pH and [H$^+$]	
pH	[H$^+$]
7.0	100.0 nmol/L*
7.1	80.0
7.2	64.0
7.3	50.0
7.4	40.0
7.5	32.0
7.6	25.0
7.7	20.0
7.8	16.0
7.9	12.5
8.0	10.0

*nmol/L = 10^{-9} M/L

Small changes in pH represent large changes in actual [H$^+$].

Note: As can be seen from the above table, a change in pH of 1 (i.e., pH of 8.0 decreasing to a pH of 7.0) represents a tenfold increase in the [H$^+$].

Small changes in pH represent _____ changes in the actual [H$^+$].

large

Note: By reviewing the above table, you can see that the normal [H$^+$] equals 40 nanomols/L. The [H$^+$] can be calculated from the following formula:

[H$^+$] = 24 × (PaCO$_2$/HCO$_3^-$)

However, as noted earlier, because of the awkwardness of expressing the actual [H$^+$], the pH is usually used instead.

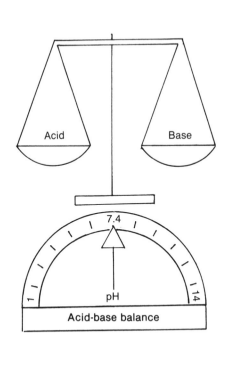

Since acids donate H^+ to a solution and bases combine with H^+ to remove them, the actual $[H^+]$ of a solution will depend on the relative proportions of acids and bases.

pH reflects the $[H^+]$ of blood and is determined by the relative proportions of _____ and _____ in the mixture.

acids, bases

If we add more H^+ (acids) to a sample of blood, its pH will _____ and it will become more acidic.

decrease

If we remove H^+ from a sample of blood, its pH will _____ and it will become less acidic.

increase

Note: We can see that blood can become more acidic from two different mechanisms: the addition of H^+ *or* the removal of bases. In the same manner, blood can become more alkaline from the removal of H^+ *or* the addition of bases.

$$pH \approx \frac{Base}{Acid} = \frac{HCO_3^-}{H_2CO_3} = \frac{24}{1.2} = \frac{20}{1}$$

It is the overall ratio of base to acid that determines the pH.

The pH of blood depends on the _____ of base to acid.

ratio

Note: The key message conveyed by the equation above is that the pH of blood depends on the ratio of base (HCO_3^-) to acid (H_2CO_3) and not by the absolute value of either one alone. When the pH of blood is 7.40, or in the middle of normal range, there are 20 parts of HCO_3^- to one part of H_2CO_3 in the blood. When this ratio is altered, the pH will change.

Disorders that upset the normal base-acid ratio in blood will cause changes in the _____.

pH

153

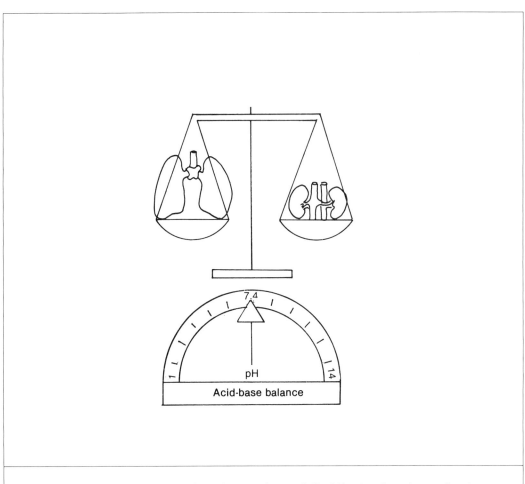

The overall pH depends on the balance between the metabolic (kidney) and respiratory (lung) functions.

We can evaluate the respiratory portion of overall acid-base balance by analyzing the _____.

$PaCO_2$

The $PaCO_2$ can be used to reflect the _____ in the blood.

$[H_2CO_3]$

We can evaluate the metabolic portion of acid-base balance by analyzing the _____.

$[HCO_3^-]$

Note: When blood gas values are determined, pH and $PaCO_2$ are measured directly by the electrodes of the blood gas machine. The value for HCO_3^- is derived by calculation. The formula utilized is called the *Henderson-Hasselbalch equation*. The calculation is based on the premise that since the pH is determined by the H_2CO_3 and HCO_3^-, when two of the three values are known, the third can be calculated.

pH = Measured

PaCO$_2$ = Measured

HCO$_3^-$ = Calculated or use nomogram

The pH and PaCO$_2$ are measured with special electrodes in the blood gas laboratory, whereas the HCO$_3^-$ value is calculated or obtained by using a nomogram.

The pH and PaCO$_2$ are directly _____ in the laboratory.   *measured*

Note: Many modern ABG-analysis devices are computerized. The PaCO$_2$, PaO$_2$, and pH are measured, but the HCO$_3^-$ value is computed using the Henderson-Hasselbalch equation. By using a special graphic device known as the Siggaard-Andersen Alignment nomogram, we can determine the HCO$_3^-$ (i.e., once we have values for pH and PaCO$_2$. See Appendix B).

If the values for pH and PaCO$_2$ are measured, the HCO$_3^-$ value may be computed or obtained by use of a _____.   *nomogram*

Normal pH = 7.40 (7.38–7.42)

The normal pH of arterial blood (pH_a) is 7.40 and is maintained within a narrow range of 7.38 to 7.42.

The pH of arterial blood is kept within the _____ limits of 7.38 to 7.42.

narrow

Note: Although pH_a is the proper symbol to denote the pH of arterial blood, the subscript *a* is usually dropped.

The normal pH is _____.

7.40

A pH value of 7.40 indicates that the overall _____ of base to acid is normal.

ratio

The normal ratio of base to acid is _____.

20 : 1

Note: Ordinarily, kidney and lung function regulate acid-base balance and keep the _____ within a relatively narrow range.

pH

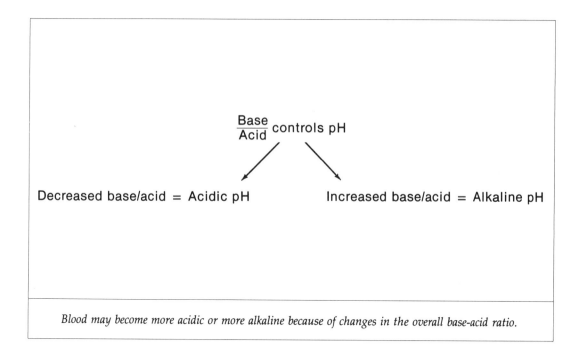

Blood may become more acidic or more alkaline because of changes in the overall base-acid ratio.

When the HCO_3^-/H_2CO_3 ratio increases to greater than 20 : 1, the pH will be _____.

alkaline

When the base-acid ratio _____ to less than 20 : 1, the pH will be acidic.

decreases

Note: Remember that it is not the absolute concentration of acid or base that ultimately determines the pH, but the relative proportions of each.

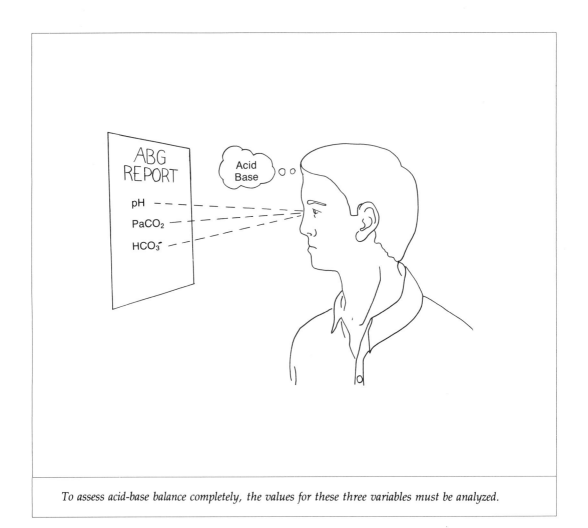

To assess acid-base balance completely, the values for these three variables must be analyzed.

The respiratory component of acid-base balance is represented by the _____.

$PaCO_2$

The metabolic component is represented by the _____ concentration.

HCO_3^-

The levels of $PaCO_2$ and HCO_3^- may vary independently, but it is the overall ratio that determines the _____.

pH

Note: The pH can be thought of as indicating the net effect of the respiratory and metabolic components (i.e., the overall balance between the two).

Systematic evaluation of acid-base status:

1. What is the overall acid-base status? pH = _____

2. What is the respiratory status? $PaCO_2$ = _____

3. What is the metabolic status? HCO_3^- = _____

When analyzing an ABG, evaluate the acid-base status from a systematic review of pH, $PaCO_2$, and HCO_3^-.

The interpretation of the acid-base status consists of a _____ review of the ABG.

systematic

List the sequence followed when analyzing the acid-base status:

☐ First, analyze the _____ .

☐ Second, analyze the _____ status.

☐ Third, analyze the _____ status.

pH
respiratory
metabolic

Note: This is the sequence that will be followed as we progress through the examples in this book.

Final step in acid-base interpretation:

4. Analysis:

   Is this an acute disorder? Chronic disorder? Simple disorder? Mixed disturbance? Combined?

   What type of compensation is occurring (if any)?

   If compensation is not as expected, does this indicate another underlying problem?

The fourth and final step in interpretation of the acid-base status is an analysis *of what the first three steps have revealed.*

The fourth step in acid-base interpretation is the _____.

analysis

Note: Analysis of the results of the first three steps is often difficult. At this point, certain clinical information about the patient may be necessary to be reasonably confident of the conclusions drawn. The first three steps are considered a "just the facts" interpretation. The last step involves considerable interpretation and integration of these facts.

1. $PaCO_2$ = _____ mmHg

2. HCO_3^- = _____ mEq/L

3. pH = _____

4. HCO_3^-/H_2CO_3 = _____

Identify the normal range of values for each of the above.

1. _____   *38 to 42*

2. _____   *22 to 26*

3. _____   *7.38 to 7.42*

4. _____   *20 : 1*

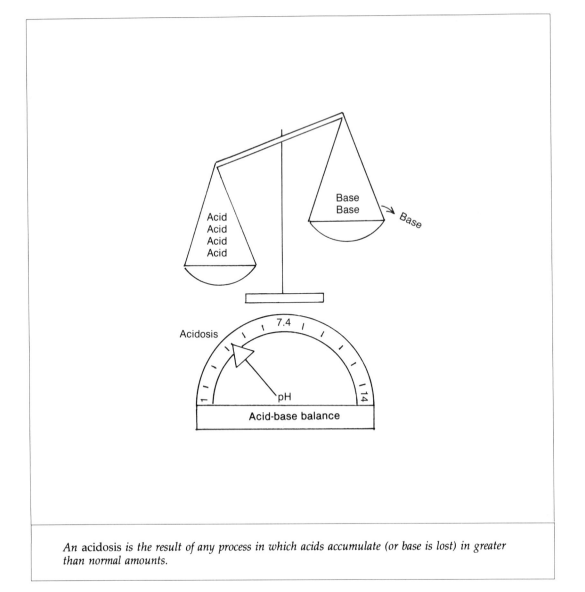

An acidosis *is the result of any process in which acids accumulate (or base is lost) in greater than normal amounts.*

Accumulation of acids is called an _____.

acidosis

An acidosis may also result from loss of _____.

base

The presence of an underlying disorder capable of producing excessive acids in the blood is referred to as an _____.

acidosis

pH<7.38 = Acidemia

If there is excessive buildup of acids in the blood causing the actual pH to be less than 7.38, the condition is called an acidemia *(acid blood).*

The lower value of the range of normal pH is _____.

7.38

When the pH is less than 7.38, the condition is called _____.

acidemia

An acidemia indicates that the overall ratio of base-acid (HCO_3^-/ H_2CO_3) has _____.

decreased

Note: An important distinction needs to be made between *acidosis* and *acidemia* (i.e., pH<7.38). An acidosis is a respiratory or metabolic condition that has the *potential* to lower the pH. Remember, the pH is the net result of the interaction between the respiratory and metabolic components. An acidosis of one component may not produce an overall base-acid ratio of less than 20 : 1 and a pH less than 7.38. The final pH will depend on what compensations occur and whether there are other acid-base disturbances.

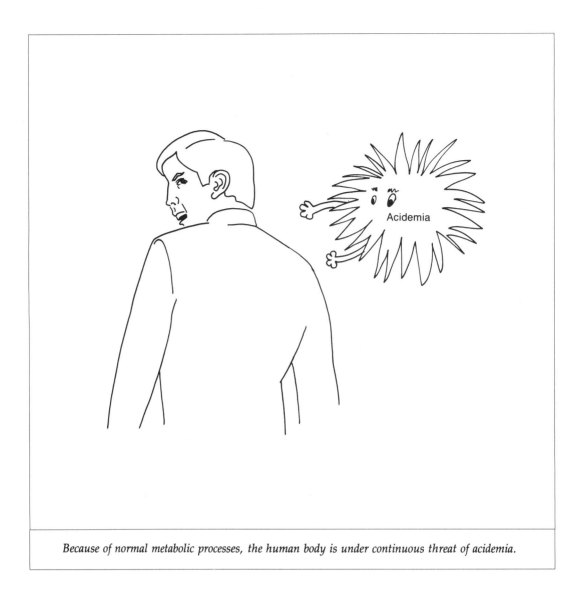

Because of normal metabolic processes, the human body is under continuous threat of acidemia.

Continuous production of _____ during normal metabolic processes poses a constant threat of acidemia.

acids

Note: The body produced 13,000 mEq of H_2CO_3 per day (from CO_2) and approximately 1 mEq per kilogram body weight of dietary acids. This accumulation would cause acidemia if this acid load were not eliminated at a rate that matched its production.

The body's daily load of acids is ultimately eliminated either by the _____ or by the _____.

lungs, kidneys

Metabolic?   Respiratory?
         pH = 7.22

                Both?

Acidemia can be of respiratory or metabolic origin or a combination of both.

An acidemic pH simply means the ratio of base-acid is
_____.   *low (<20 : 1)*

If acidemia is of metabolic origin, the level of HCO_3^- in the blood
will be _____.   *low*

If acidemia is of respiratory origin, then the low base-acid ratio is
being caused by an increased _____ level, reflected in   *acid or H_2CO_3*
an elevation of $PaCO_2$.

Sometimes acidemia is due to a combination of both metabolic
and respiratory _____ occurring at the same time and   *acidosis*
independently of each other (i.e., mixed acidosis).

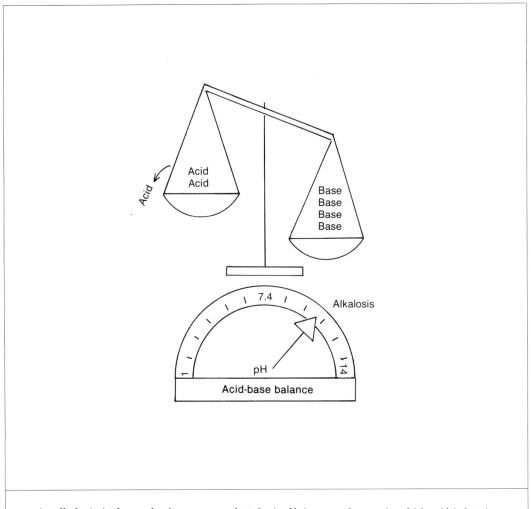

An alkalosis *is the result of any process that, by itself, increases base or in which acid is lost in greater than normal amounts.*

An alkalosis will result when there is accumulation of greater than normal amounts of _____.

base

Excessive loss of _____ will also cause an alkalosis.

acids

Note: Individual respiratory or metabolic components alone do not determine the final pH. The important point to remember is that two or more acid-base disorders may coexist, each capable of changing one part of the ratio, but which cumulatively cancel out the effects of each other, with the net result that there is little or no change in the overall base-acid ratio. For example, an alkalosis in one component (respiratory or metabolic) may not cause the pH to increase if there is coexisting acidosis in the other component.

pH>7.42 = Alkalemia

If there is an excessive accumulation of base causing the final pH of the blood to be greater than 7.42, the condition is called alkalemia *(alkaline blood).*

An increase in the base-acid ratio will cause the pH to _____.   *increase*

When the blood pH is greater than 7.42, the condition is called _____.   *alkalemia*

An acid-base change that can potentially cause a pH greater than 7.42 is referred to as an _____.   *alkalosis*

pH = 7.55 ?

?   ?   ?   ?
Respiratory?   Metabolic?

Combined?

Alkalemia may be respiratory or metabolic in origin or both.

Alkalemia simply means the base-acid ratio of the blood is
_____.

high (>20 : 1)

Alkalemia that is associated with an elevated _____ indicates that the disorder is metabolic in origin (i.e., metabolic alkalosis).

HCO_3^-

Alkalemia that results from a low $PaCO_2$ means that the disorder is _____ in origin (i.e., respiratory alkalosis).

respiratory

When alkalemia is associated with a high level of HCO_3^- and a
low $PaCO_2$ occurring at the same time, we are dealing with a
mixed metabolic and respiratory _____.

alkalosis

pH = 7.60?

Metabolic?   Respiratory?

Combined?

The pH alone does not identify the source of an acid-base imbalance.

In the above example, the pH is high, which indicates the blood is _____.

alkalemic

The origin of the alkaline pH may be respiratory, _____, or both.

metabolic

Although the base-acid ratio is _____, we cannot determine from the pH alone whether it is due to a high amount of base (metabolic alkalosis), a low amount of acid (respiratory alkalosis), or _____.

high

both

1. pH = 7.31

2. pH = 7.41

3. pH = 7.49

Describe the acid-base condition of the blood in each of the above pHs.

1. _____   *acidemia*

2. _____   *normal*

3. _____   *alkalemia*

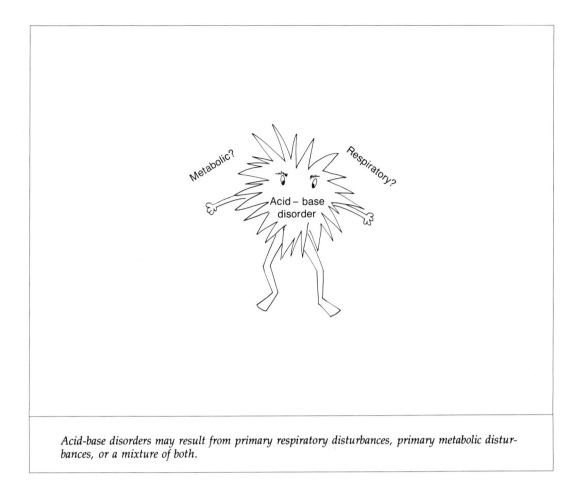

Acid-base disorders may result from primary respiratory disturbances, primary metabolic disturbances, or a mixture of both.

An acid-base disturbance in which the primary abnormality involves a disturbance in the concentration of H_2CO_3 (i.e., change in the $PaCO_2$) is referred to as a _____ acid-base disorder.

respiratory

A disturbance in which the primary abnormality is reflected in a change in the HCO_3^- concentration is referred to as a _____ acid-base disorder.

metabolic

If the primary problem involves both respiratory and metabolic components, we are dealing with a _____ acid-base disturbance.

mixed

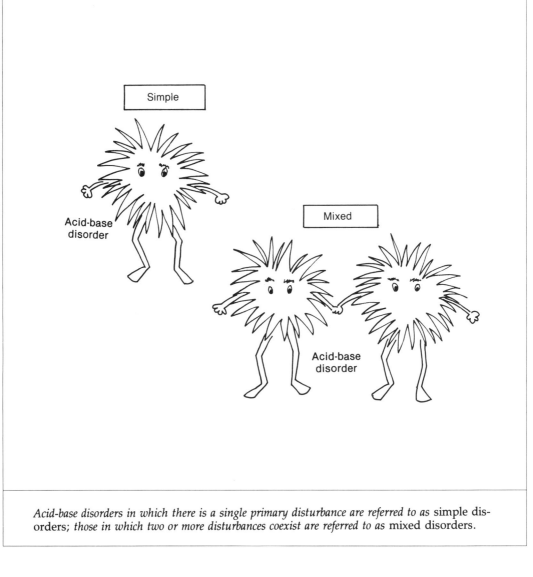

Acid-base disorders in which there is a single primary disturbance are referred to as simple dis-orders; *those in which two or more disturbances coexist are referred to as* mixed disorders.

In a simple disorder, only _____ primary acid-base disturbance exists.

one

In a _____ disorder, there is a combination of acid-base disturbances.

mixed

Note: When dealing with mixed acid-base disorders, an analysis of the parameters obtained from the ABG alone may sometimes completely fail to reflect the extent or nature of the various acid-base disorders present. In these cases, data obtained from other sources such as examination of the patient, laboratory tests, and clinical history are often needed to clarify the nature of the disturbance.

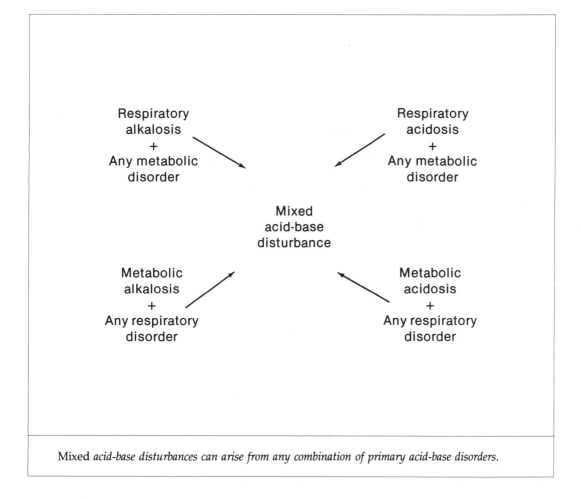

Mixed *acid-base disturbances can arise from any combination of primary acid-base disorders.*

A mixed acid-base disturbance occurs when there is a _____ of primary respiratory and metabolic disorders.

combination

Note: When we refer to mixed disorders, we mean that there is more than one primary acid-base problem. If the ABG values are consistent with a single primary disorder with normal expected compensation, then we are dealing with a simple rather than a mixed disorder. For example, the combination of a primary metabolic acidosis and a compensatory respiratory alkalosis (i.e., a normal expected compensatory response to the primary disorder) would *not* be termed a mixed disorder.

In mixed disorders, there is more than one _____ disturbance in the acid-base balance.

primary

Note: If the primary metabolic and respiratory disorders in a mixed acid-base disturbance are both acidotic or alkalotic, we sometimes use the term *combined* interchangeably with *mixed* (e.g., combined respiratory and metabolic acidosis).

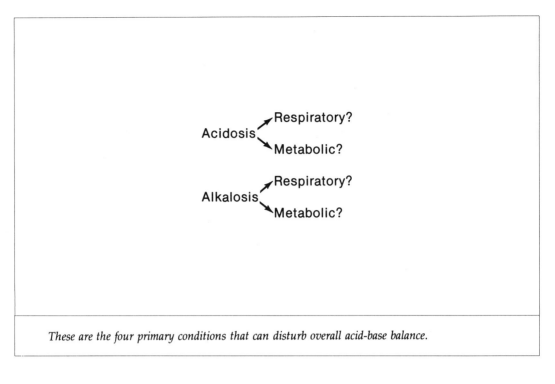

These are the four primary conditions that can disturb overall acid-base balance.

Acidosis can be of respiratory or _____ origin, or both.   *metabolic*

Alkalosis can be of metabolic or _____ origin or both.   *respiratory*

When the primary disturbance involves changes in [H_2CO_3] (i.e., change in the $PaCO_2$), we are dealing with a _____ acid-base disorder.   *respiratory*

A metabolic acid-base disorder is one in which the primary abnormality involves changes in the _____ level.   *HCO_3^-*

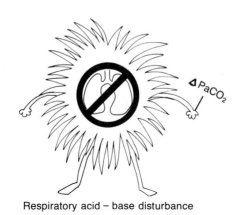

Respiratory acid – base disturbance

Respiratory acid-base disturbances are characterized by changes in the PaCO$_2$.

The respiratory system regulates the PaCO$_2$ through changes in
_____ ventilation.   *alveolar*

Acid-base disorders of _____ origin are reflected by   *respiratory*
changes in the PaCO$_2$.

To determine if we are dealing with a respiratory acid-base disorder, we must check the _____.   *PaCO$_2$*

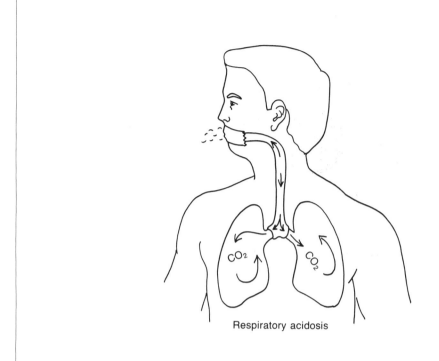

Respiratory acidosis

In primary respiratory acidosis, there is buildup of CO_2 in the blood because of inadequate removal by the lungs (i.e., hypoventilation).

Hypoventilation will lead to a buildup of _____ in the blood.

CO_2

Retention of CO_2 causes an acid-base disturbance known as respiratory _____.

acidosis

A patient who has a high $PaCO_2$ is said to be _____.

hypoventilating

Note: When the retention of CO_2 in the blood (i.e., $PaCO_2 > 42$ mmHg) is due to abnormal functioning of the respiratory system, it is known as a *primary* respiratory acidosis. If the retention of CO_2 is due to the body's attempt to compensate for a metabolic acid-base disturbance, it is known as a *compensatory* respiratory acidosis. Although the high $PaCO_2$ is in both cases referred to as a respiratory acidosis, it does not always represent a primary disturbance in acid-base balance.

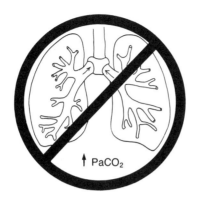

Primary respiratory acidosis has many causes, but the common denominator is failure of the respiratory system to remove adequate amounts of CO_2.

Respiratory acidosis is the acid-base disturbance in which CO_2 elimination through the lungs is _____.

inadequate

The common underlying problem in respiratory acidosis is that the lungs do not eliminate adequate amounts of _____.

CO_2

Note: Primary respiratory acidosis may result from any condition that impairs alveolar ventilation. This includes both pulmonary and nonpulmonary problems such as central nervous system depression, respiratory muscle weakness, upper airway obstruction, primary lung disease, and chest wall disorders. Severe chronic obstructive pulmonary disease is the most common cause of primary respiratory acidosis.

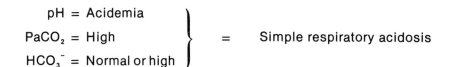

$$pH = \text{Acidemia}$$
$$PaCO_2 = \text{High}$$
$$HCO_3^- = \text{Normal or high}$$
$$\Big\} = \text{Simple respiratory acidosis}$$

When acidemia is caused exclusively by retention of CO_2, we are dealing with simple respiratory acidosis.

Note: In a simple disorder, the acidotic or alkalotic process will result in acidemia or alkalemia, respectively. On the other hand, in a mixed disorder the combination of acidotic or alkalotic processes may or may not result in acidemia or alkalemia, depending on the relative intensity of the primary disorders.

In simple respiratory acidosis, the acid-base disturbance is caused exclusively by a rise in the _____.

PaCO₂

In simple respiratory acidosis, the pH is _____.

low

When acidemia arises from an increase in $PaCO_2$ rather than a fall in $[HCO_3^-]$, the primary disorder is _____ in origin.

respiratory

Note: In simple respiratory acidosis the $[HCO_3^-]$ may be normal *or* high depending on the lack of, or presence of, metabolic compensation. When evaluating any acid-base disorder, it is important to determine the nature and extent of compensations expected in response to a primary change in the respiratory or metabolic components of acid-base balance. Any deviations from these expected responses may signal the presence of either a second primary disturbance or presence of a mixed acid-base disorder. (See pp. 198–202 for more on expected compensations.)

$$pH = 7.25$$
$$PaCO_2 = 58 \text{ mmHg}$$
$$HCO_3^- = 25 \text{ mEq/L}$$

What does the above ABG demonstrate?

The pH indicates an _____.   *acidemia*

The $PaCO_2$ is increased, indicating a respiratory _____.   *acidosis*

The HCO_3^- value is within _____ limits.   *normal*

This appears to be a _____ respiratory acidosis.   *simple*

Note: The presence of a normal $[HCO_3^-]$ implies a lack of compensation. Either the primary respiratory disorder has occurred very recently, resulting in inadequate time for compensation to occur, or there is a kidney problem preventing expected compensation. This observation should be discussed during the analysis stage of the ABG interpretation.

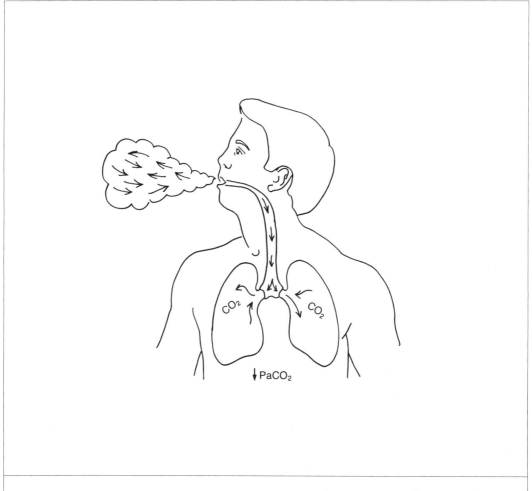

Primary respiratory alkalosis refers to the acid-base disorder in which the elimination of CO_2 by the lungs is excessive (i.e., hyperventilation).

_____, or excessive ventilation, will result in an acid-base disorder known as respiratory alkalosis.

Hyperventilation

When hyperventilation occurs, CO_2 is being excessively removed by the lungs and the $PaCO_2$ falls below _____ mmHg.

38

When too much CO_2 is eliminated by the lungs, the resulting acid-base disorder is known as _____ alkalosis.

respiratory

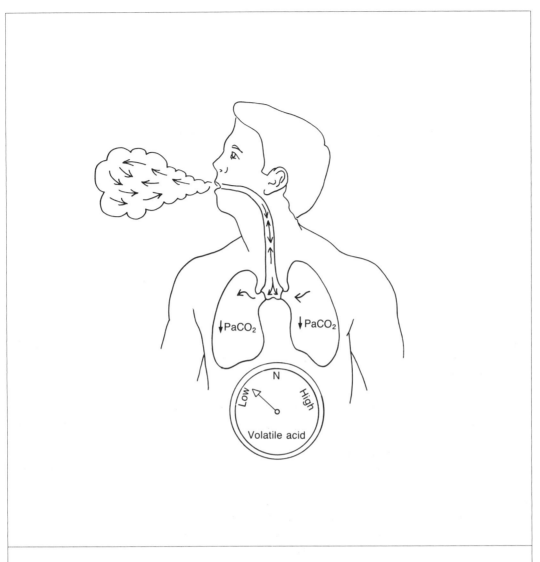

When CO_2 is eliminated excessively, the $PaCO_2$ is low and there is a fall in the normal quantities of volatile acid.

In respiratory alkalosis, excessive CO_2 elimination by the lungs results in a low _____ .

$PaCO_2$

When CO_2 is eliminated excessively, there is a fall in the amount of volatile _____ acid.

carbonic

Note: Remember, a reduction in H_2CO_3 may be due to a primary respiratory acid-base disorder (i.e., a primary respiratory alkalosis) or it may be an adaptive response to the accumulation of excess metabolic acids in the body (i.e., a compensatory respiratory alkalosis).

```
pH      = Alkalemia     ⎫
PaCO₂   = Low           ⎬  = Simple respiratory alkalosis
HCO₃⁻   = Normal or low ⎭
```

Alkalemia caused exclusively by a low PaCO₂ is referred to as a simple respiratory alkalosis.

Since alkalemia can be either respiratory or _____ in origin (or both), we must look at the $PaCO_2$ and $[HCO_3^-]$ to determine which is the cause.

metabolic

If the $PaCO_2$ is low and the $[HCO_3^-]$ is normal or low, the alkalemia must be _____ in origin.

respiratory

A combination of a high pH, a low $PaCO_2$, and a normal or low $[HCO_3^-]$ is called a simple respiratory _____.

alkalosis

Note: Ordinarily, the kidneys compensate for a respiratory acid-base imbalance. The absence of such an adaptive response usually means there has not been enough time for compensation and we are dealing with an *acute* respiratory acid-base disorder. The alternate explanation for a normal $[HCO_3^-]$ in this situation is the presence of a kidney disorder preventing compensation.

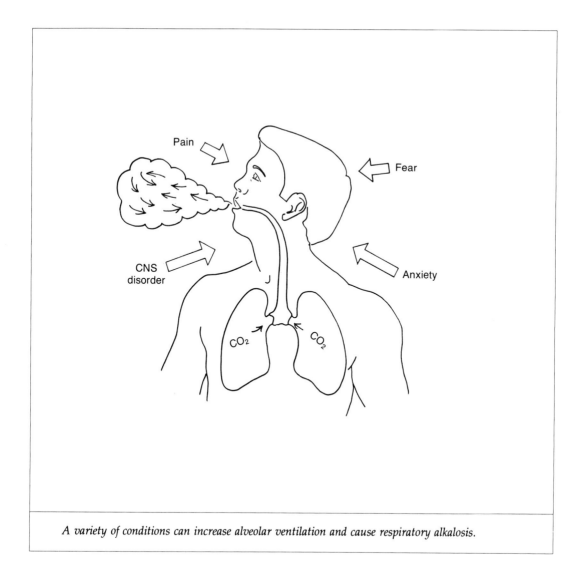

A variety of conditions can increase alveolar ventilation and cause respiratory alkalosis.

Respiratory alkalosis results from excessive _____ ventilation.

alveolar

Hyperventilation is recognized by a fall in the $PaCO_2$ below _____ mmHg.

38

Note: Hyperventilation leading to excessive removal of CO_2 is seen in a variety of disorders that may be of pulmonary or non-pulmonary origin. These include central nervous system disorders, primary lung disorders, toxic metabolic problems, anxiety, mechanical overventilation, and acute blood loss. Hyperventilation also occurs as a compensatory response to metabolic acidosis.

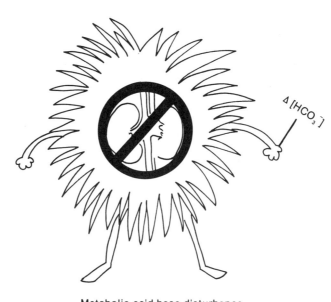

Metabolic acid-base disturbance

Metabolic acid-base disturbances are characterized by changes in the $[HCO_3^-]$.

The level of HCO_3^- in the blood is regulated by the _____.

kidneys

An acid-base disorder in which the primary abnormality involves the level of HCO_3^- is referred to as a _____ disorder.

metabolic

Note: A disturbance in the HCO_3^- level may occur as a result of a primary metabolic acid-base disorder, or it may represent a compensatory response to a primary respiratory acid-base disorder.

Metabolic acidosis = $[HCO_3^-] < 22$ mEq/L

Metabolic acidosis is an acid-base disorder that results in an abnormally low level of HCO_3^- ($[HCO_3^-] < 22$ mEq/L).

In metabolic acidosis, the $[HCO_3^-]$ is less than _____.

22mEq/L

When an acid-base disorder is _____ in origin, it is re-flected by a change in the level of HCO_3^-.

metabolic

A disorder leading to a low blood level of HCO_3^- is referred to as metabolic _____.

acidosis

Note: Even though a low $[HCO_3^-]$ defines a metabolic acidosis, keep in mind there are really two types of metabolic acidosis. In primary metabolic acidosis, the low $[HCO_3^-]$ is attributable to a disorder of the metabolic system, whereas in compensatory metabolic acidosis the $[HCO_3^-]$ is low in order to compensate for a primary respiratory alkalosis.

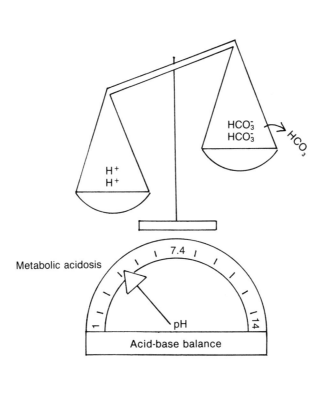

Primary metabolic acidosis can result from either a loss of HCO_3^- or an increase in the amount of $[H^+]$ from accumulation of nonvolatile acid(s).

Disease processes in which HCO_3^- is lost will cause primary metabolic _____.

acidosis

Primary metabolic acidosis may also result from processes that increase the blood level of _____ acids.

nonvolatile

Note: Whatever the underlying cause, the body responds to an increase in nonvolatile acid by using the base HCO_3^- to combine with the acid to protect itself. As a result, blood levels of HCO_3^- will be low. Regardless of cause, the hallmark of metabolic acidosis is a low $[HCO_3^-]$.

pH   = Acidemia
PaCO$_2$ = Normal or low $\Big\}$ = Simple metabolic acidosis
HCO$_3^-$ = Low

When acidemia is caused exclusively by a low [HCO$_3^-$], we are dealing with a simple metabolic acidosis.

A low blood pH indicates the presence of _____.

acidemia

The combination of a low pH and low [HCO$_3^-$] with a normal or low PaCO$_2$, indicates that the acidemia is _____ in origin.

metabolic

Note: In the presence of metabolic acidemia, the PaCO$_2$ would be expected to be low as the body attempts to compensate and prevent any further decline in pH. If the PaCO$_2$ is normal or high, very serious problems with the respiratory system exist and the question must be raised: Why can't this patient hyperventilate as expected with the stimulus of the acidemia? In these cases, an abnormality of the respiratory system must be suspected.

In simple metabolic acidosis, the PaCO$_2$ would be expected to be _____.

low

$$pH = 7.30$$
$$PaCO_2 = 40 \text{ mmHg}$$
$$HCO_3^- = 19.2 \text{ mEq/L}$$

Analyze the above ABG data.

The pH is low, which indicates _____.   *acidemia*

The PaCO$_2$ level is _____.   *normal*

The low [HCO$_3^-$] tells us the acidemia is _____ in origin.   *metabolic*

Note: In the presence of acidemia, the normal level of PaCO$_2$ is disturbing. Although at first glance we may be tempted to call this a simple metabolic acidosis, there appears to be a second problem present. The inability of the body to compensate for metabolic acidosis by blowing off CO$_2$ indicates a respiratory problem.

Metabolic alkalosis = [HCO$_3^-$]>26 mEq/L

Metabolic alkalosis is an acid-base imbalance that results in an abnormally high level of HCO$_3^-$ ([HCO$_3^-$] > 26 mEq/L).

Metabolic alkalosis is indicated by a _____ level of HCO$_3^-$.

high

A [HCO$_3^-$] greater than _____ mEq/L indicates a metabolic alkalosis.

26

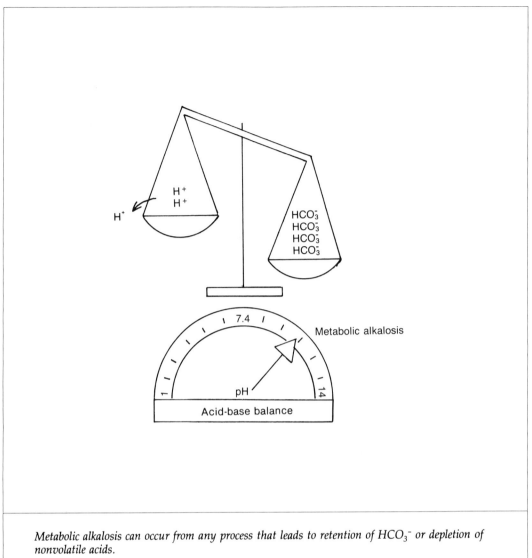

Metabolic alkalosis can occur from any process that leads to retention of HCO_3^- or depletion of nonvolatile acids.

Any process that leads to retention of _____ will cause a metabolic alkalosis.

HCO_3^-

Loss of nonvolatile _____ causes a metabolic alkalosis.

acids

Note: A depletion of nonvolatile acids causes a relative excess of HCO_3^-. As H^+ is removed (along with the nonvolatile acid), HCO_3^- is released into the blood. Remember, an increase in HCO_3^- can result from an underlying disease process (in which case it is referred to as a primary metabolic alkalosis) or as a compensatory response to a primary respiratory acidosis (in which case it is referred to as a compensatory metabolic alkalosis).

$$
\left.
\begin{array}{l}
\text{pH} \quad = \text{Alkalemia} \\
\text{PaCO}_2 = \text{Normal or high} \\
\text{HCO}_3^- = \text{High}
\end{array}
\right\} = \text{Simple metabolic alkalosis}
$$

When alkalemia is caused exclusively by a high HCO_3^-, we are dealing with a simple *metabolic alkalosis.*

If there is alkalemia and the $[HCO_3^-]$ is high while the $PaCO_2$ is normal or high, we know the alkalemia must be _____ in origin.

metabolic

Alkalosis caused exclusively by a metabolic disorder is referred to as a _____ metabolic alkalosis.

simple

Note: Since the respiratory compensation for a metabolic disorder will occur very rapidly, we cannot infer how long a metabolic disorder has existed from the lack or presence of respiratory compensation. As a result, it is difficult to use the labels *acute* or *chronic* in reference to metabolic disorders without knowledge of previous ABGs or the patient's history. (See pp. 198–202, 218–225 for further discussion of the expected respiratory compensation.)

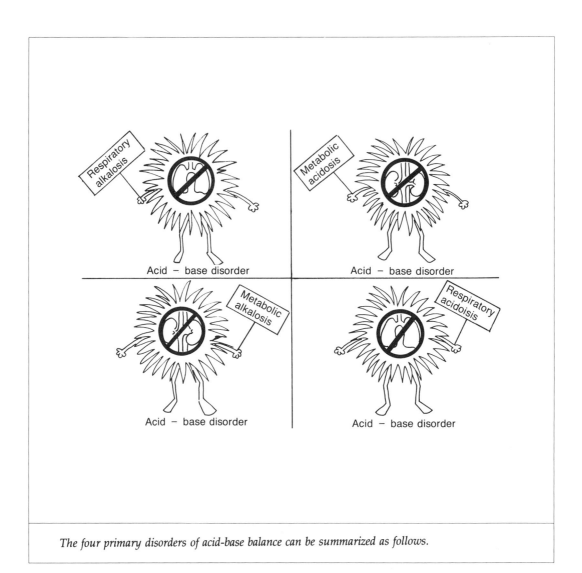

Acid – base disorder

Acid – base disorder

Acid – base disorder

Acid – base disorder

The four primary disorders of acid-base balance can be summarized as follows.

When the basic disorder causes a decrease in $PaCO_2$, we call this a primary respiratory _____.

alkalosis

When the basic disorder causes an increase in $[HCO_3^-]$, we call this a primary metabolic _____.

alkalosis

When the basic disorder causes a decrease in $[HCO_3^-]$, we call this a primary metabolic _____.

acidosis

When the basic disorder causes an increase in $PaCO_2$, we call this a primary respiratory _____.

acidosis

Note: Remember, if the change in $PaCO_2$ or $[HCO_3^-]$ is the result of a compensatory action by the body, it is not referred to as a primary alkalosis or acidosis.

Primary acid-base disturbances:?

List the four types of primary acid-base disturbances.

1. _____
2. _____
3. _____
4. _____

respiratory acidosis
respiratory alkalosis
metabolic acidosis
metabolic alkalosis

See Table 5-1 on page 246 to review the common causes of simple acid-base disorders.

pH

Chemical buffering→|7.38–7.42|←Physiologic compensations

There are two fundamental ways in which the body responds to threats to acid-base balance and attempts to maintain pH within normal limits.

Defense of pH is accomplished in _____ ways.   *two*

Despite daily threats to acid-base balance, the body tries to maintain _____ within a narrow range.   *pH*

The body protects itself against changes in pH by chemical _____ and by physiologic _____.   *buffering, compensations*

Note: Threats to acid-base balance are normally handled by chemical buffers that react immediately to minimize change in pH. In addition to buffer mechanisms, additional adaptations occur whenever the primary disorder persists for any length of time. Physiologic compensation by the lungs for metabolic imbalance usually occurs rapidly (within minutes), whereas physiologic compensation by the kidneys for respiratory imbalance may take from hours to a few days.

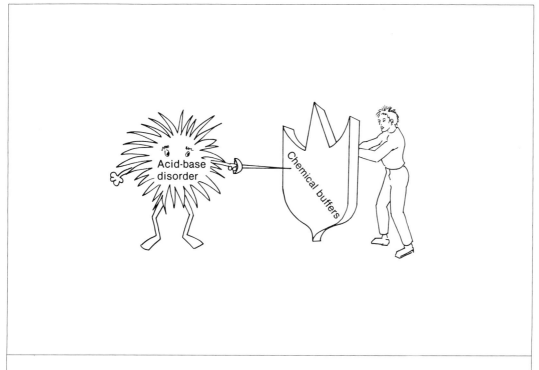

Chemical buffers act as the first line of defense in protecting the body fluids against disturbances in acid-base balance.

Note: Buffers are substances that lessen or absorb some of the shock of a sudden change or impact. In dealing with acid-base balance, a buffer may be regarded as a chemical ''sponge.'' Depending on the particular acid-base disturbance, a buffer can soak up or release excess H^+ to minimize fluctuations of pH. In the language of chemistry, a buffer system consists of a weak acid in combination with one of the salts of that acid (a base). Although there are many buffer systems in the body, the most important one is the HCO_3^- buffer system, which consists of sodium bicarbonate (base) and H_2CO_3. Disturbances in acid-base balance will upset the normal ratio of HCO_3^-/H_2CO_3 of 20 : 1.

Buffers do not prevent the change in pH from occurring. Rather, they reduce the amount or magnitude of the change that would have occurred if they had not been present.

Chemical buffers help minimize changes in the _____ of the blood.

pH or [H⁺]

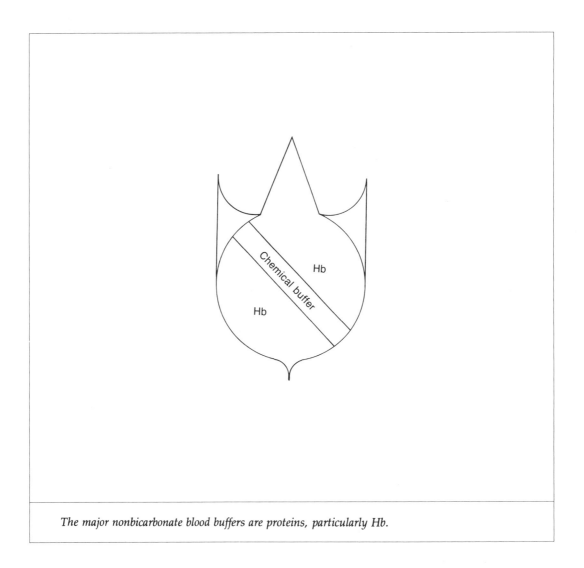

The major nonbicarbonate blood buffers are proteins, particularly Hb.

In addition to the HCO_3^-/H_2CO_3 buffer system, the blood is buffered by _____.

proteins

Note: Proteins and HCO_3^- each make up approximately half of the total blood buffer level. However, the HCO_3^-/H_2CO_3 buffer system is an "open" system in that its volatile acid (i.e., H_2CO_3) can be eliminated through alveolar ventilation. Moreover, the kidneys control its other component (i.e., HCO_3^-). Consequently, HCO_3^-/H_2CO_3 is considered the blood's most important buffer system.

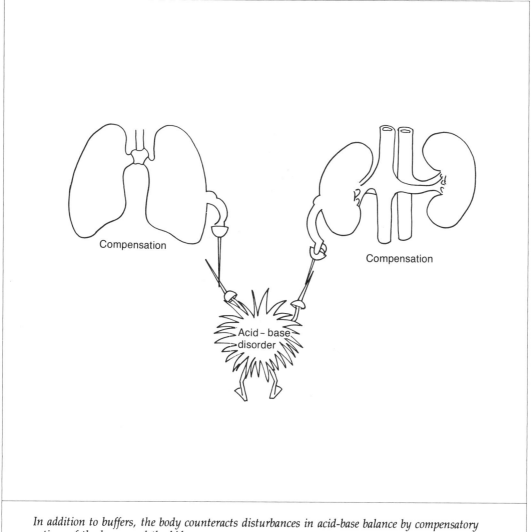

Compensation

Compensation

Acid – base disorder

In addition to buffers, the body counteracts disturbances in acid-base balance by compensatory actions of the lungs and the kidneys

Acid-base disturbances are normally handled by blood buffers and physiologic compensations by the _____ and the _____.

kidneys
lungs

The chemical _____ systems act as the first line of defense until compensatory mechanisms can come into play.

buffer

Buffer mechanisms are chemical reactions that are called into play _____ following a challenge to acid-base balance.

immediately

Subsequently, compensatory actions of the kidney and lung may attempt to restore the normal _____ of the base-acid and return the pH toward normal.

ratio

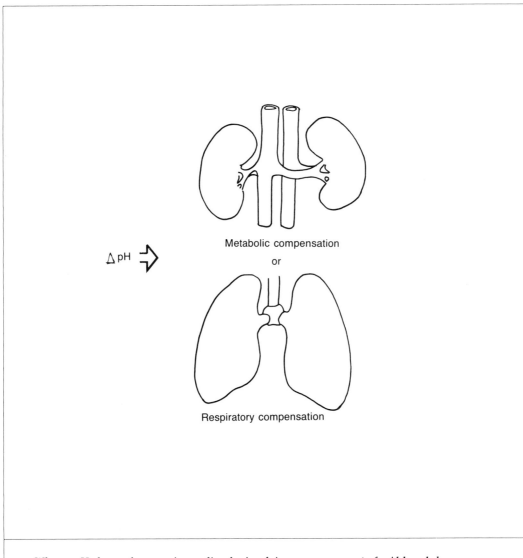

Δ pH

Metabolic compensation

or

Respiratory compensation

When a pH change from a primary disorder involving one component of acid-base balance occurs, physiologic compensation usually involves the other component.

Note: For example, a primary respiratory alkalosis will induce a retention of acid by the kidneys, sometimes referred to as a compensatory metabolic acidosis. In addition to acid retention, the kidneys will increase excretion of HCO_3^- in an attempt to bring the base-acid ratio back toward a normal 20 : 1.

A primary metabolic disorder will induce physiologic compensation by the _____ system.

respiratory

A primary respiratory disorder will induce compensation by the _____ component of acid-base balance.

metabolic

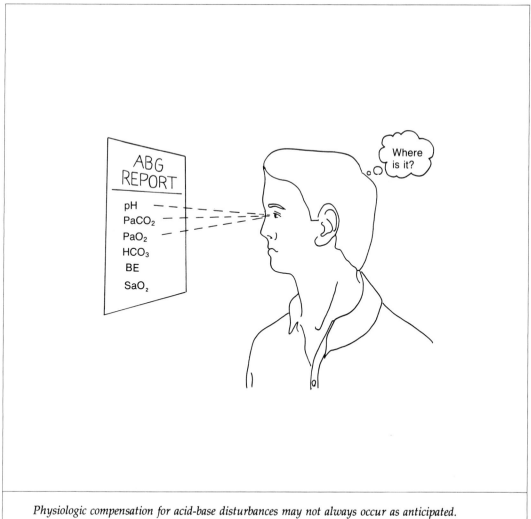

Physiologic compensation for acid-base disturbances may not always occur as anticipated.

The metabolic component does not always compensate for primary _____ acid-base problems.

respiratory

Note: Sometimes this is due to lack of adequate time to compensate. In other cases, it is due to the presence of a second primary acid-base disorder. It can also be due to a primary problem with kidney function resulting in inability to compensate (e.g., kidney disease).

The respiratory system does not always compensate for primary _____ disturbances.

metabolic

Note: Frequently a patient's failure to compensate for metabolic acidosis by increasing the level of ventilation is due to underlying lung disease.

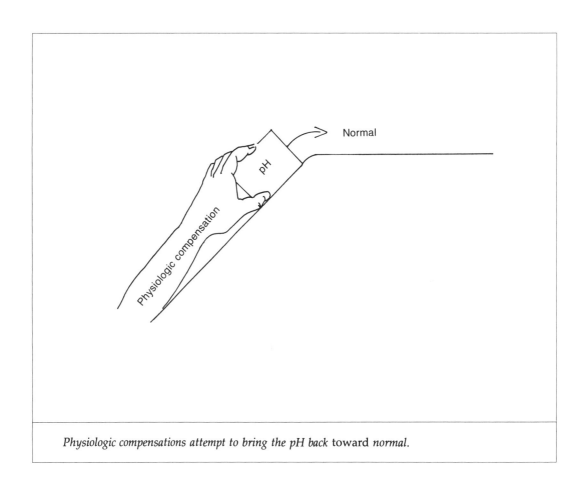

Physiologic compensations attempt to bring the pH back toward normal.

Although compensatory responses to primary acid-base disorders attempt to restore normal values, the pH will still be
_____.

abnormal

In the presence of a single primary acid-base disorder, even after compensation has occurred the _____ will still be displaced in the direction of the primary disorder.

pH

If a patient has primary respiratory acidosis with metabolic compensation, the pH will still be _____.

acidic

If a patient has primary metabolic acidosis with respiratory compensation, the pH will still be _____.

acidic

If a patient has primary respiratory alkalosis with metabolic compensation, the pH will still be _____.

alkaline

If a patient has primary metabolic alkalosis with respiratory compensation, the pH will still be _____.

alkaline

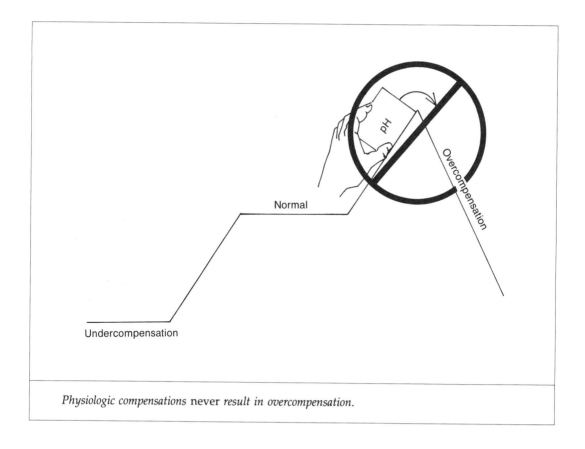

Physiologic compensations never *result in overcompensation.*

Physiologic compensations to acid-base disturbances _____ result in overcompensation.

never

Note: An example of overcompensation would be if a primary respiratory acidosis were followed by so much metabolic compensation that the pH becomes alkalotic (see example below). This does not make physiologic sense and does not happen. If there is overcorrection of the pH, then we are dealing with a second primary acid-base disorder. Consider the following ABG:

pH = 7.46

$PaCO_2$ = 56 mmHg

HCO_3^- = 40 mEq/L

If the increase in HCO_3^- represented metabolic compensation for respiratory acidosis, it would be demonstrating so much HCO_3^- retention that the pH would be brought from an acidic value, past a normal pH, to the point of being alkaline. This simply does not occur. When the observed values lie outside expected levels of compensation, we are probably dealing with a second primary acid-base disorder (or we have misinterpreted the results and need to reanalyze the data).

Primary disorder	Physiologic compensation
Respiratory acidosis	Kidney—retention of HCO_3^-; excretion of H^+
Respiratory alkalosis	Kidney—excretion of HCO_3^-; retention of H^+
Metabolic acidosis	Lung—excretion of H^+ (CO_2)
Metabolic alkalosis	Lung—possible retention of H^+(CO_2)

The physiologic compensation anticipated in response to each of the primary acid-base disorders can be summarized as follows.

Primary metabolic acidosis causes _____ compensation consisting of increased ventilation and a fall in _____.

respiratory
$PaCO_2$

Primary metabolic alkalosis may cause _____ compensation in which ventilation decreases and there is a small rise in the $PaCO_2$.

respiratory

Primary respiratory acidosis leads to _____ compensation, which consists of a rise in the kidney excretion of H^+ and retention of HCO_3^-.

metabolic

Primary respiratory alkalosis causes metabolic compensation consisting of H^+ retention through the kidney and increased excretion of _____.

HCO_3^-

Note: The expected degree of compensation and the time it takes to achieve that compensation will vary with each primary disturbance. The following pages describe in more detail the anticipated compensation for each of the primary acid-base disorders.

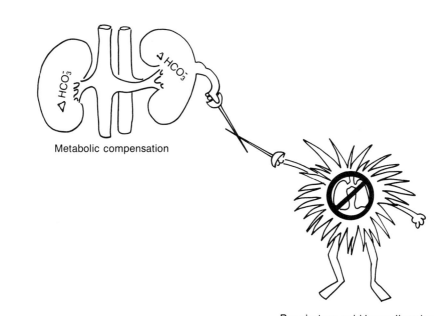

Metabolic compensation

Respiratory acid-base disorder

In response to respiratory acid-base disorders, the kidneys alter their HCO_3^- resorption; this is called metabolic compensation.

A respiratory acid-base abnormality will usually cause _____ compensation.

metabolic

Metabolic compensation is accomplished by alteration of _____ resorption of HCO_3^-.

kidney

The alteration of HCO_3^- resorption through the kidneys begins within hours but can take several days to exert its _____ effect.

maximum

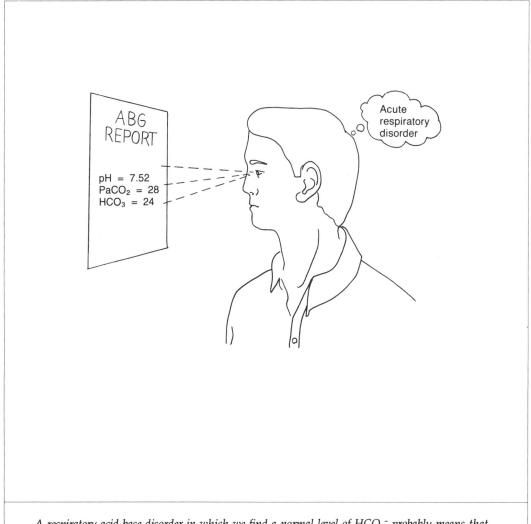

A respiratory acid-base disorder in which we find a normal level of HCO_3^- probably means that the disturbance is acute.

A respiratory disorder in which the HCO_3^- is normal usually means the disorder is _____.

acute

Often the lack of compensation means there has not been enough _____ for the kidneys to respond; hence this is probably an acute disturbance.

time

Note: Although the absence of metabolic compensation usually implies that the respiratory acid-base disturbance is acute, in some cases it may imply the presence of a kidney disorder. In such cases, there may be a problem with the kidneys that prevents them from doing their usual job of metabolic compensation.

$$pH = 7.33$$
$$PaCO_2 = 50 \text{ mmHg}$$
$$HCO_3^- = 25.8 \text{ mEq/L}$$

What would the above ABG data indicate?

The low blood pH indicates an _____.   *acidemia*

Since the $PaCO_2$ is high and the $[HCO_3^-]$ is normal, the acidemia
is due to a primary _____ acidosis.   *respiratory*

The patient's metabolic status is _____.   *normal*

Because of the normal $[HCO_3^-]$, this respiratory acid-base disorder could be interpreted as being _____.   *acute*

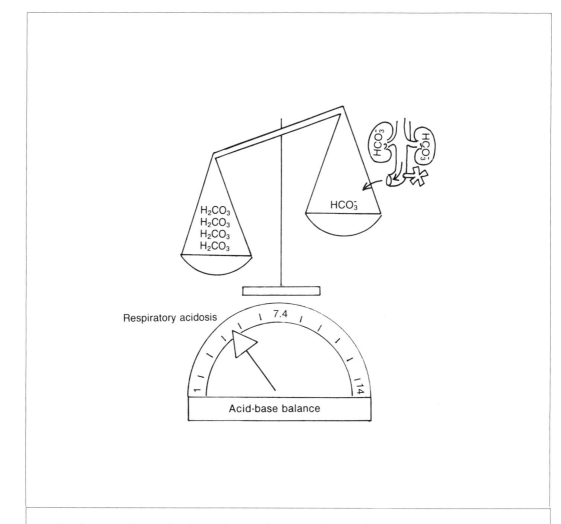

A primary respiratory disorder can be termed acute *or* chronic *depending on the lack or presence of a compensatory metabolic response.*

An increase in PaCO$_2$ is also known as respiratory _____.   *acidosis*

Respiratory acidosis will usually cause _____ compensation.   *kidney or metabolic*

In rapidly developing respiratory acidosis, the base-acid ratio will initially _____ as a result of the increase in the PaCO$_2$ (i.e., volatile H$_2$CO$_3$).   *fall*

To bring the ratio back toward a normal value of _____, the kidneys will _____ resorption of HCO$_3^-$.   *20 :1*
                    increase

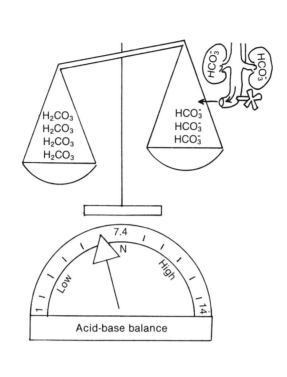

Of all the physiologic acid-base compensations, the kidney's retention of HCO_3^- to balance an increase in H_2CO_3 is the most nearly complete (i.e., the pH is brought back to near normal levels).

The metabolic compensation for respiratory acidosis leads to an increase in HCO_3^- that nearly matches the increase in _____ associated with the primary disorder.

H_2CO_3

Although the metabolic compensation to respiratory acid-base disorders can be nearly _____, it usually takes several days to achieve.

complete

When respiratory acidosis is sustained for several days, metabolic compensation may bring the _____ back to a near normal level.

pH

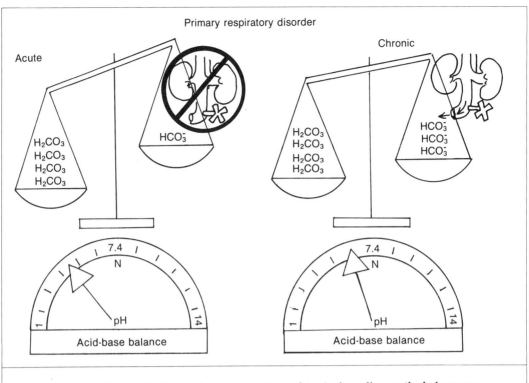

A primary respiratory disorder can be termed acute *or* chronic *depending on the lack or presence of a compensatory metabolic response.*

The term acute means that there has not been enough _____ for the compensatory response.

time

An acute respiratory disorder may show no signs of metabolic _____.

compensation

Metabolic compensation for respiratory disorders usually takes hours to begin and several _____ to complete.

days

The absence of metabolic compensation to a primary respiratory acid-base disorder (i.e., [HCO₃⁻] is normal while PaCO₂ is high or low) infers that we are probably dealing with an _____ disturbance.

acute

In primary respiratory acidosis, if there is marked elevation of the PaCO₂ but the pH is only slightly acidotic, we can infer that the disorder is probably _____.

chronic

Note: Since respiratory compensation for a primary metabolic disorder occurs very quickly, the presence or lack of compensation is not useful in determining the length of time the acid-base disorder has existed.

$$pH = 7.25$$
$$PaCO_2 = 60 \text{ mmHg}$$
$$HCO_3^- = 25.5 \text{ mEq/L}$$

Does the above ABG imply that the respiratory disorder is acute or chronic?

The pH is decreased, so we have an _____.   *acidemia*

Since the $PaCO_2$ is high and the $[HCO_3^-]$ is normal, the acidemia
is due to a primary _____ acidosis.   *respiratory*

Since the $[HCO_3^-]$ is still _____, it is apparent that   *normal*
there is no metabolic _____.   *compensation*

We are probably dealing with an _____ disorder.   *acute*

Note: Rapid increases in $PaCO_2$ may cause a dramatic fall in pH
(i.e., acidemia). This is referred to as an acute respiratory acidosis. The terms *acute* and *uncompensated* are often interchanged.

Acute?   Chronic?

$$pH = 7.37$$
$$PaCO_2 = 56\,mmHg$$
$$HCO_3^- = 33\,mEq/L$$

This ABG was just handed to you. Do you think this is an acute or a chronic disorder?

The pH is nearly _____.   *normal*

The elevated $PaCO_2$ indicates a respiratory _____.   *acidosis*

The kidneys have apparently increased resorption of _____, HCO_3^-
bringing the pH back toward normal.

It appears we are dealing with a _____ respiratory   *chronic*
acidosis.

Rule number 1: For every acute PaCO₂ *increase* of 15 mmHg (above 35 mmHg), expect the [HCO₃⁻] to *increase* by 1 mEq/L.

Rule number 2: For every acute PaCO₂ *decrease* of 5 mmHg (below 35 mmHg), expect the [HCO₃⁻] to *decrease* by 1 mEq/L.

Although [HCO₃⁻] changes are primarily related to changes in the metabolic status, acute changes in PaCO₂ also cause small predictable changes in the [HCO₃⁻].

Note: We have already referred to the interactions among CO_2, H_2O, H_2CO_3, HCO_3^-, and H^+:

$$CO_2 + H_2O \leftrightharpoons H_2CO_3 \leftrightharpoons H^+ + HCO_3^-$$

From the above equation, we can see that large increases or decreases in CO_2 will produce predictable changes in [HCO₃⁻]. The above rules of thumb can be applied whenever a patient's PaCO₂ is significantly above or below normal.

If a patient's PaCO₂ acutely increases to 65 mmHg, you would expect the [HCO₃⁻] to increase by _____ mEq/L.

2

If a patient's PaCO₂ acutely falls to 25 mmHg, you would expect the [HCO₃⁻] to _____ by 2 mEq/L.

decrease

Note: The above guidelines should help you realize that in certain instances (e.g., with large PaCO₂ changes) slight changes in the level of HCO₃⁻ may be of respiratory origin and are not always representative of metabolic changes.

```
Base excess (BE) ≈ Metabolic component
```

Since [HCO_3^-] can be influenced by changes in PaCO_2 (even if only slightly), some prefer to use base excess (BE)* as the indicator of the metabolic component.

Note: BE is another method of describing the metabolic status of a patient. It reflects a relative increase or decrease in a patient's buffer base level. The normal value is between -2 and $+2$ mEq/L. Using this method, a BE less than -2 (e.g., -5) indicates a deficit of base and hence is referred to as a *base deficit* (i.e., metabolic acidosis). A BE greater than $+2$ indicates an excess of base (i.e., metabolic alkalosis). This method helps to quantify the degree of metabolic imbalance. There are, however, problems with using blood BE. Problems arise because the total extracellular fluid (ECF) compartment as well as intracellular buffers are involved with buffering and the BE of blood does not accurately represent the total buffering of the body. Consequently, despite alternatives, we prefer using the $[HCO_3^-]$ to give us a simple and reasonably accurate estimation of the metabolic status. One must remember, however, to keep in mind the influence of large PaCO_2 changes on the $[HCO_3^-]$ (as described on p. 211).

Although BE can be used to evaluate the metabolic status, _____ is reasonably accurate and probably simpler to use.

$[HCO_3^-]$

*Refers to BE of blood.

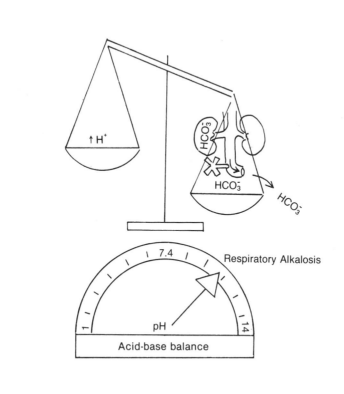

In chronic respiratory alkalosis, the kidneys compensate by decreasing H⁺ excretion and increasing HCO₃⁻ excretion.

Chronic respiratory alkalosis usually results in _____ compensation by the kidneys.

metabolic

In chronic respiratory alkalosis, HCO₃⁻ excretion is _____, resulting in metabolic compensation.

increased

Note: With persistence of respiratory alkalosis beyond several days, the increase in HCO₃⁻ excretion is due to the fact that there is decreased resorption taking place in the kidneys. Renal compensation also results in decreased H⁺ loss.

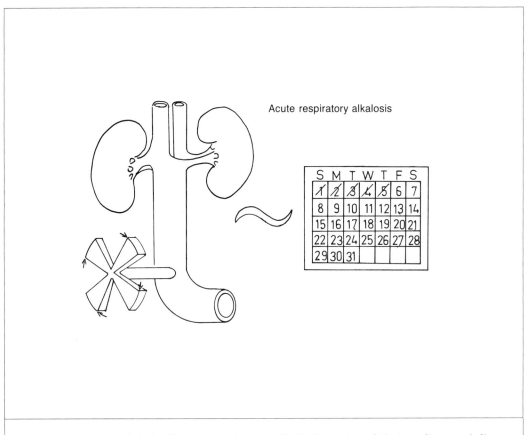

Acute respiratory alkalosis

Acute respiratory alkalosis (like acute respiratory acidosis) does not result in immediate metabolic compensatory responses.

Note: In respiratory alkalosis, the metabolic compensation by the kidneys may take hours to begin and several days to complete. In contrast to the metabolic compensation for respiratory acidosis, the compensation for respiratory alkalosis is less complete, less predictable, and often results in only *partial compensation*. Partial compensation is defined as a compensatory response that brings the pH back toward normal but does not reach it.

A rapid decrease in $PaCO_2$ will cause an _____ in pH.

increase

In the absence of any metabolic compensation, the rapid fall in $PaCO_2$ will result in acute _____.

alkalemia

Partial compensation means the pH has been brought back only part way _____ normal.

toward

$$pH = 7.50$$

$$PaCO_2 = 30 \text{ mmHg}$$

$$HCO_3^- = 23.4 \text{ mEq/L}$$

Does this acid-base disorder appear to be acute or chronic?

The high blood pH indicates an _____.

alkalemia

The combination of a high pH, low $PaCO_2$ and normal $[HCO_3^-]$ tells us we are dealing with a primary respiratory _____.

alkalosis

The normal $[HCO_3^-]$ indicates an absence of any metabolic _____.

compensation

This lack of compensation implies that the respiratory alkalosis is _____.

acute

$$pH = 7.34$$

$$PaCO_2 = 60 \text{ mmHg}$$

$$HCO_3^- = 32.3 \text{ mEq/L}$$

What level of compensation does this ABG reflect?

The low blood pH indicates an _____.

acidemia

The high $PaCO_2$ indicates a respiratory _____.

acidosis

The pH, $PaCO_2$ and $[HCO_3^-]$ values tell us that the high $[HCO_3^-]$ probably represents metabolic _____ for a primary respiratory acidosis.

compensation

The degree of compensation appears to be _____.

partial

Note: It is possible that given more time, the kidneys may compensate further. It is also possible that sufficient time has elapsed and that the kidneys have reached their limit and are unable to increase HCO_3^- retention further.

$$pH = 7.55$$

$$PaCO_2 = 25 \text{ mmHg}$$

$$HCO_3^- = 21.5 \text{ mEq/L}$$

What do think of this ABG?

The blood pH is markedly elevated indicating there is severe
_____ .   *alkalemia*

The low $PaCO_2$ indicates a respiratory _____ .   *alkalosis*

Note: Keep in mind the $PaCO_2$'s small effect on $[HCO_3^-]$ before
determining the metabolic status (if you are confused, review p.
211).

The $[HCO_3^-]$ indicates a _____ metabolic status (once   *normal*
the slight drop in $[HCO_3^-]$ from the low $PaCO_2$ is accounted for,
the $[HCO_3^-]$ is accepted as normal).

This ABG could be interpreted as an _____ respiratory   *acute*
alkalosis.

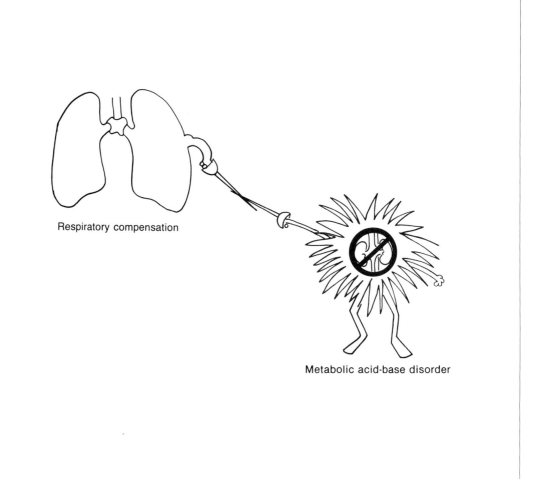

Respiratory compensation

Metabolic acid-base disorder

In reaction to primary metabolic acid-base disorders, there are adaptive ventilatory responses that will affect the level of CO_2 in the blood. This adaptation is called respiratory compensation.

An imbalance in the metabolic acid-base status causes _____ compensation.

respiratory

Respiratory compensation is accomplished by increasing or decreasing alveolar _____.

ventilation

As alveolar ventilation changes, the _____ level and, hence, the H_2CO_3 level changes.

CO_2

Note: As noted earlier, the respiratory response to metabolic disturbance usually occurs within minutes. Because of the rapid response to metabolic imbalance, it is often not possible to determine if a metabolic disorder is acute or chronic by the presence of respiratory compensation.

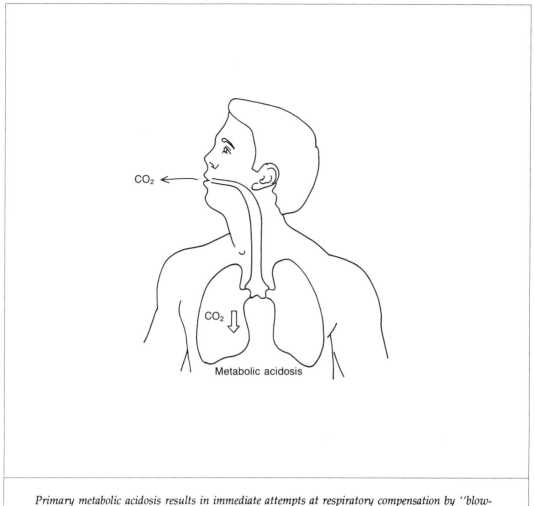

CO₂ ←

CO₂ ⇓

Metabolic acidosis

Primary metabolic acidosis results in immediate attempts at respiratory compensation by "blowing off" CO_2.

An increase in the [H⁺] in the blood stimulates the respiratory control center, leading to an increase in _____.

ventilation

As ventilation increases, more CO_2 is "blown off" and the $PaCO_2$ _____.

falls

By blowing off CO_2, the lungs are actually reducing the level of _____ in the blood.

H_2CO_3 or acid

Note: The nature of this response is highly predictable. For every decrease in the [HCO_3^-] of 1 mEq/L, the $PaCO_2$ generally falls by approximately 1 mmHg.

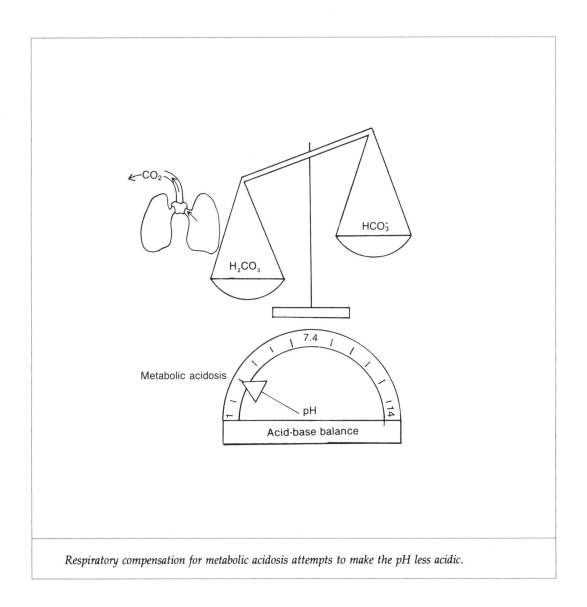

Respiratory compensation for metabolic acidosis attempts to make the pH less acidic.

Metabolic acidosis _____ the base-acid ratio, causing the pH to _____.

lowers
decrease

In metabolic acidosis, the base-acid ratio is low because of a fall in _____.

HCO_3^- *or base*

In response to metabolic acidosis, respiratory compensation reduces the level of _____ by blowing off CO_2 gas.

H_2CO_3

Note: In metabolic acidosis, the $[HCO_3^-]$ is low. In this case, blowing off CO_2 and thereby reducing the H_2CO_3 will increase the base-acid ratio and bring it back toward 20 : 1. If a metabolic acidosis is of sufficient magnitude to reduce the pH to approximately 7.20, the respiratory compensation would be expected to raise the pH halfway back toward normal, or to about 7.30.

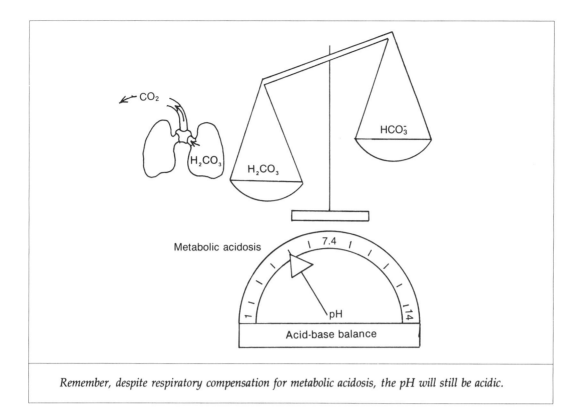

Remember, despite respiratory compensation for metabolic acidosis, the pH will still be acidic.

Despite respiratory compensation, the pH remains _____ during a metabolic acidosis.

low or acidic

Note: In the presence of metabolic acidosis, the lungs will not normally excrete enough H_2CO_3 to bring the pH all the way back to normal. The low pH provides a continued stimulus to hyperventilate.

Acidemia _____ the respiratory center and leads to respiratory compensation.

stimulates

Note: The normal expected degree of respiratory compensation may be easily recognized by inspection of the last two digits of the pH and the $PaCO_2$. If these numbers are close, the respiratory response is appropriate. For example:

pH	Expected $PaCO_2$
7.25	25
7.30	30
7.35	35

Of course, this rule of thumb is only approximate but it does aid in quick recognition of "appropriate" respiratory compensation. This rule is valid down to a pH of approximately 7.20.

$$pH = 7.31$$

$$PaCO_2 = 29.5 mmHg$$

$$HCO_3^- = 14.5\ mEq/L$$

Evaluate this patient's acid-base status and the respiratory response to metabolic acidosis.

The low blood pH indicates the presence of _____.

acidemia

In response to the acidemia, the patient is hyperventilating as evidenced by the low _____.

PaCO₂

The combination of the low $[HCO_3^-]$ and the low $PaCO_2$ indicates that the acidemia must be due to a primary _____ acidosis.

metabolic

The $PaCO_2$ of 29.5 is numerically close to 31 (last two digits of the pH). This appears to be an _____ respiratory response.

appropriate or normal

$$pH = 7.41$$

$$PaCO_2 = 23 \text{ mmHg}$$

$$HCO_3^- = 14.4 \text{ mEq/L}$$

What do you think about this patient's response to metabolic acidosis?

The blood pH is _____.   *normal*

The $PaCO_2$ indicates a respiratory _____.   *alkalosis*

The $[HCO_3^-]$ indicates a metabolic _____.   *acidosis*

Note: One way to interpret the above data is to conclude that we are dealing with a primary metabolic acidosis with complete respiratory compensation. However, we know that normal expected compensation to a primary disorder rarely brings the pH back to a completely normal value. Consequently, we should look for some other reason for this degree of hyperventilation, as this is not likely to be just a normal respiratory compensation. Based on what we know about compensations, this patient appears to have a primary respiratory alkalosis in addition to a primary metabolic acidosis.

On the other hand, the above ABG could also be interpreted as showing complete metabolic compensation for a respiratory alkalosis (which is, of course, also not likely to occur). It should be obvious why it is not always possible to correctly interpret some ABGs without additional data on the patient!

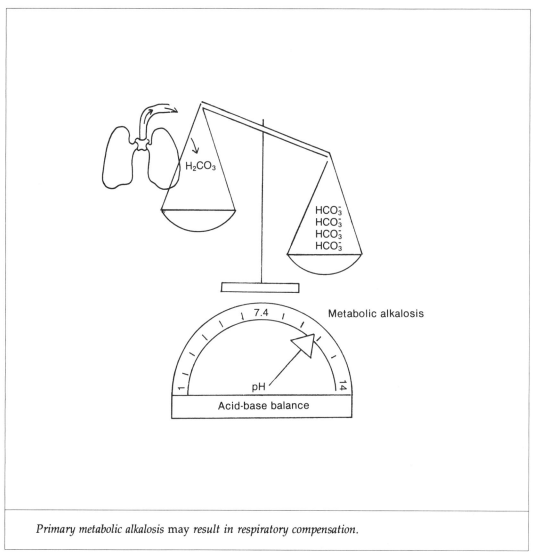

Primary metabolic alkalosis may *result in respiratory compensation.*

Metabolic alkalosis is recognized by an increased _____.

HCO_3^-

Note: Small increases in blood $[HCO_3^-]$ are usually not associated with changes in ventilation (i.e., $PaCO_2$).

In response to metabolic alkalosis, there may be respiratory

_____.

compensation

Respiratory compensation for metabolic _____ is not considered as predictable, as it is for metabolic acidosis.

alkalosis

Note: With so many inputs to your respiratory center to keep you breathing, a slight alkalemia from a metabolic alkalosis usually will not depress your ventilation.

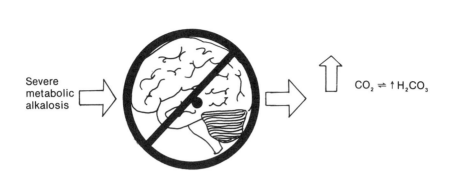

Severe metabolic alkalosis → CO₂ ⇌ ↑H₂CO₃

$CO_2 \rightleftharpoons \uparrow H_2CO_3$

Severe degrees of metabolic alkalosis may result in mild suppression of the respiratory center with retention of CO_2 and elevation of H_2CO_3.

Ordinarily, mild degrees of metabolic alkalosis are not associated with changes in _____.

PaCO₂ or ventilation

When the degree of metabolic alkalosis is _____, there may be respiratory compensation in the form of hypoventilation causing retention of CO_2.

severe

Note: As a general rule, for every increase in the serum $[HCO_3^-]$ of 1 mEq/L over 40 mEq/L there may be an equivalent increase in the $PaCO_2$ of 1 mmHg. It is rare for respiratory compensation to be such that the $PaCO_2$ rises above 50 mmHg.

See Table 5-2 on page 247 to review recognition of simple acid-base disorders.

$$pH = 7.59$$

$$PaCO_2 = 46.5 \text{ mmHg}$$

$$HCO_3^- = 45 \text{ mEq/L}$$

What is your interpretation of the acid-base status of this ABG?

The high blood pH indicates an _____.   *alkalemia*

The respiratory status indicates a respiratory _____.   *acidosis*

The elevated [HCO_3^-] indicates a metabolic _____.   *alkalosis*

The slight hypoventilation appears to be a _____ re-   *compensatory*
sponse to the severe metabolic alkalosis.

Note: Remember, respiratory compensation for metabolic alkalosis is neither very efficent nor reliable. This amount of compensation is probably typical for this degree of alkalemia.

See Table 5-3 on page 247 to review expected compensation in
simple acid-base disorders.

Primary metabolic acidosis

       +   = Severe acidemia

Primary respiratory acidosis

When primary respiratory acidosis and primary metabolic acidosis coexist, the result is usually severe acidemia.

Respiratory acidosis that occurs at the same time as metabolic acidosis is known as a _____ disorder.

mixed

This can also be referred to as a _____ metabolic and respiratory acidosis.

combined

These two coexisting disturbances often result in severe _____.

acidemia

Note: A patient who develops metabolic acidosis and is unable to respond and hyperventilate to blow off CO_2 is in serious trouble. This severe disorder is usually seen in critically ill patients and requires immediate attention.

pH = 7.23

$PaCO_2$ = 58 mmHg

HCO_3^- = 18 mEq/L

You are handed the ABG above. What do you think about the acid-base status?

The blood pH is low, indicating an _____.   *acidemia*

The patient is hypoventilating as evidenced by the high
_____.   *$PaCO_2$*

The high $PaCO_2$ means there is a respiratory _____.   *acidosis*

However, the [HCO_3^-] is low, which means there is also a metabolic _____.   *acidosis*

This patient has a _____ respiratory and metabolic aci-   *mixed or combined*
dosis and is in serious trouble.

Primary respiratory alkalosis

                    +   = Severe alkalemia

Primary metabolic alkalosis

Combined respiratory and metabolic alkalosis can result in dangerous alkalemia.

When both the respiratory and the metabolic components are alkalotic, the condition is termed a _____ respiratory and metabolic alkalosis.

combined

With two primary disorders, this may also be called a _____ acid-base disturbance.

mixed

Note: A pH greater than approximately 7.60 is considered a very serious threat to the patient. Severe alkalemia can result in dangerous cardiac arrhythmias as well as interfere with the function of the nervous system.

$$pH = 7.62$$

$$PaCO_2 = 28 \text{ mmHg}$$

$$HCO_3^- = 29.2 \text{ mEq/L}$$

What is your acid-base interpretation of this ABG?

The high blood pH indicates an _____.   *alkalemia*

The $PaCO_2$ demonstrates a _____ alkalosis.   *respiratory*

The $[HCO_3^-]$ indicates a metabolic _____.   *alkalosis*

This patient's severe alkalemia is the result of a combined respiratory and metabolic _____.   *alkalosis*

Note: This patient has a life-threatening alkalemia that requires immediate attention.

$$pH = 7.39$$
$$PaCO_2 = 64 \text{ mmHg}$$
$$HCO_3^- = 39 \text{ mEq/L}$$

When an ABG appears to demonstrate complete physiologic compensation, consider the possibility of a mixed disturbance.

The blood pH is _____.   *normal*

The high $PaCO_2$ tells us that there is a respiratory _____.   *acidosis*

The [HCO_3] demonstrates a metabolic _____.   *alkalosis*

Note: Although the ABG above is consistent with a compensatory metabolic response for chronic respiratory acidosis, it could also be seen in a patient with acute respiratory acidosis (e.g., sudden respiratory depression from a drug overdose) who has a second primary disturbance (metabolic alkalosis). In this case, the two primary acid-base disorders balance each other and result in a normal pH. This dilemma demonstrates why the complete interpretation of a single ABG often requires correlation with clinical or other data (e.g., comparison with prior ABGs).

The above ABG could be the result of a _____ acid-base disturbance.   *mixed*

$$pH = 7.42$$

$$PaCO_2 = 52 \text{ mmHg}$$

$$HCO_3^- = 34.5 \text{ mEq/L}$$

The analysis stage of acid-base interpretation can be very difficult. What is your acid-base interpretation of the above ABG?

The blood pH is _____.

normal

The high $PaCO_2$ indicates a respiratory _____.

acidosis

The _____ $[HCO_3^-]$ tells us there is a metabolic alkalosis.

high

If we interpret the $PaCO_2$ and $[HCO_3^-]$ values as representing respiratory compensation for a primary metabolic alkalosis, they would be demonstrating _____ compensation (and we already know that this is not likely to occur).

complete

If, on the other hand, we interpret the $PaCO_2$ and $[HCO_3^-]$ values as representing metabolic compensation for a primary respiratory acidosis, they would be demonstrating _____ (and we know that this is also not likely to occur).

overcompensation

Note: Without more information, interpretation of this ABG is difficult. The analysis stage of acid-base interpretation often requires more information than that provided by a single ABG, particularly when trying to distinguish between a mixed disturbance and a primary disturbance with a strong compensatory response.

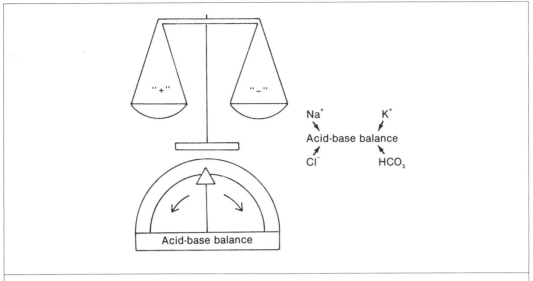

The plasma concentration of different electrolytes is very important in relationship to acid-base balance.

Note: The blood contains various positively and negatively charged ions, which must be maintained in electrical neutrality (i.e., the total number of positive charges [cations] is exactly counterbalanced by the number of negative charges [anions]). To demonstrate this electrical neutrality would require that measurements be made of all circulating charged ions. Rather than carry out exhaustive and unnecessary analysis of all cations and anions in the plasma, electrolyte tests routinely measure only sodium (Na^+), potassium (K^+), chloride (Cl^-), and bicarbonate (HCO_3^-). The serum Na^+ and K^+ account for 95 percent of the plasma cations, whereas CL^- and HCO_3^- account for 85 percent of the anions.

Positively charged electrolytes or ions are known as _____.   *cations*

The two major cations of the plasma are _____ and K^+.   *Na^+*

Negatively charged ions are known as _____.   *anions*

The major anions of plasma are HCO_3^- and _____.   *Cl^-*

Note: The normal value for the electrolytes routinely measured are as follows (all values in mEq/L).

Na^+	K^+	Cl^-	HCO_3^-
132–142	3.5–5.0	98–106	22–26

$$\text{Anion gap} = (\text{Na}^+ + \text{K}^+) - (\text{Cl}^- + \text{HCO}_3^-)$$

Normally, the sum of anions measured on an electrolyte analysis does not fully counterbalance the sum of the measured cations: their difference, expressed in mEq/L, is termed the anion gap.

Note: We know that all positive charges must be neutralized by an equal number of negative charges. Therefore, the *anion gap* simply means that anions other than Cl^- and HCO_3^- must be present to counterbalance the remainder of the combined positive charge of Na^+ and K^+.

Although the plasma concentration of individual anions or cations may vary, their sum must always be _____.

equal

The _____ gap is estimated from the difference in concentration between the measured plasma cations and anions.

anion

Note: Since the serum K^+ concentration is low and fairly constant, the equation more commonly used to calculate the anion gap is as follows:

$$\text{Anion gap} = (\text{Na}^+) - (\text{Cl}^- + \text{HCO}_3^-)$$
$$= 140 - (103 + 24)$$
$$= 13 \text{ mEq/L}*$$

*Normal range is approximately 10 to 16 mEq/L.

Note: The addition of strong organic acids, other than hydrochloric acid (HCl), to body fluids will affect the electrolyte pattern. The H^+ from the acid will convert HCO_3^- to H_2CO_3, which, as a volatile acid, is eliminated by the lungs as CO_2 gas. This loss of HCO_3^- not only leads to acidosis but also represents a loss of anions, which were balancing the positive charges. This loss of anions (from the decreased HCO_3^-) is offset by an increase in anions generated from the acid. Since these additional anions will not be measured on the routine electrolyte analysis, this leads to an increase in the calculated anion gap.

Metabolic acidosis is recognized by a fall in the serum _____.

HCO_3^-

The increase in anions associated with the addition of acids to the body causes an _____ in the anion gap.

increase

Note: When metabolic acidosis is caused by addition of HCl or loss of HCO_3^- from the body fluids, the fall in HCO_3^- is offset by a rise in the concentration of Cl^- and the anion gap remains unaltered. This is referred to as *normal anion gap metabolic acidosis.*

Electrolyte	1 (mEq/L)	2 (mEq/L)
Na^+	140	142
Cl^-	113	103
HCO_3^-	15	15
Anion gap	?	?

The above sets of electrolyte values are handed to you. Calculate the anion gaps.

In sample 1, the anion gap is _____ mEq/L.

12

In this case, the decrease in HCO_3^- is balanced by an increase in _____, resulting in a normal anion gap.

Cl^-

In sample 2, the anion gap is _____ mEq/L.

24

Addition of strong acids to the body, which results in a rise in unmeasureable anions, causes the anion gap to _____.

increase

Causes of metabolic acidosis	
Increased anion gap	Normal anion gap

Exogenous addition of acids
  Salicylates
  Methanol
	Primary HCO_3^- loss
	  From GI tract: severe diarrhea, ileostomy, colostomy

Increased metabolic acid formation
  Diabetic keto acid
  Uremic acid
  Lactic acid
	From kidneys: renal tubular acidosis
	
	Addition of acids with Cl^-
	  Hydrochloric acid
	  Ammonium chloride

The anion gap can be used to assist in the evaluation of metabolic acidosis.

Metabolic acidosis associated with an _____ anion gap occurs when there is accumulation of organic acids as in lactic acidosis or ketoacidosis.

increased

Metabolic acidosis associated with a _____ anion gap is usually attributable to loss of HCO_3^- or administration of an acid containing Cl^-.

normal

In uremic acidosis or in acidosis caused by ingestion of methanol, the anion gap is _____.

increased

When metabolic acidosis is due to a primary loss of HCO_3^-, the associated increase in _____ will result in a normal anion gap.

Cl^-

$$pH = 7.24$$

$$PaCO_2 = 26 \text{ mmHg} \qquad Na^+ = 141 \text{ mEq/L}$$

$$PaO_2 = 106 \text{ mmHg} \qquad Cl^- = 102 \text{ mEq/L}$$

$$HCO_3^- = 11.0 \text{ mEq/L}$$

Interpret the above ABG. Include your assessment of the anion gap.

The PaO_2 indicates that arterial oxygenation is _____. *adequate*

The patient is hyperventilating, as indicated by the low

_____. *PaCO₂* — *PaCO$_2$*

The increase in PaO_2 approximates the decrease in $PaCO_2$; thus
the A-aDO_2 is _____. *normal*

The low blood pH indicates an _____. *acidemia*

The $PaCO_2$ is low, indicating respiratory _____. *alkalosis*

The HCO_3^- value of 11 mEq/L indicates a metabolic _____. *acidosis*

Since the pH is acidemic, the low $PaCO_2$ appears to be _____ *compensation*
for a primary metabolic acidosis.

The anion gap is _____ mEq/L, indicating that there is *28*
an increased anion gap metabolic acidosis.

Note: This ABG and electrolytes were obtained from a diabetic
patient who had not been taking insulin for several days and developed diabetic ketoacidosis.

See Table 5-4 on page 247 to review ABG interpretation.

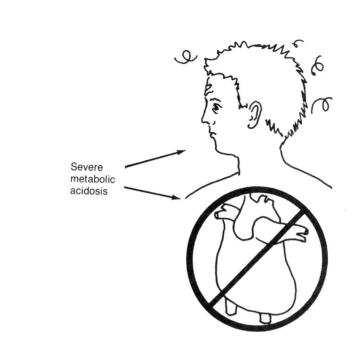

Severe
metabolic
acidosis

When severe metabolic acidosis (pH < 7.2, HCO$_3^-$ < 15 mEq/L) is associated with life-threatening cardiovascular or neurologic abnormalities, urgent elevation of the blood HCO$_3^-$ is indicated.

Note: In cases of severe metabolic acidosis, rapid elevation of the blood HCO$_3^-$ is best accomplished by administration of sodium bicarbonate (NaHCO$_3$). The amount of HCO$_3^-$ to be given may be estimated by multiplying the desired change in plasma [HCO$_3^-$] by 40 percent of the body weight measured in kilograms, (i.e., the distribution of HCO$_3^-$ is generally about 40% of the body weight). The total HCO$_3^-$ deficit may be estimated by the following formula:

HCO$_3^-$ deficit (in mEq)

= (body weight in kg) (0.40) [(desired [HCO$_3^-$])

− (measured [HCO$_3^-$])]

Note: To avoid overcorrection, one-half the calculated deficit is usually replaced. After administering HCO$_3^-$, an ABG should be rechecked to assess the results of therapy.

Once the deficit of HCO$_3^-$ is calculated, _____ of this amount is usually administered.

one-half

$$pH = 7.22$$
$$PaCO_2 = 35 \text{ mmHg}$$
$$PaO_2 = 86 \text{ mmHg}$$
$$HCO_3^- = 14 \text{ mEq/L}$$

An ABG taken from an acutely ill 60-kg-man reveals the above data. What dose of HCO_3^- should be given to correct his metabolic acidosis?

Note: The desired HCO_3^- used in the equation to calculate the appropriate HCO_3^- deficit is usually presumed to be 24 mEq/L.

The total deficit in this situation is _____ mEq/L.   *240*

Since we usually give one-half the calculated deficit, the HCO_3^- dose should be _____ mEq/L.   *120*

After giving HCO_3^-, the _____ should be rechecked to assess the effects of therapy and to reevaluate acid-base balance.   *ABG*

Note: Here is the calculation of the deficit if you need to review:

Total HCO_3^- deficit $= (60) \times (0.40) \times (24 - 14)$
$= 240$ mEq.

```
                    ABG No. 1
                    pH = 7.18              Na⁺ = 140 mEq/L

                  PaCO₂ = 25 mmHg          Cl⁻ =  94 mEq/L

                   PaO₂ = 38 mmHg

                   HCO₃⁻ = 9 mEq/L
```

This set of electrolytes and ABG No. 1 were obtained from a 70-kg-man with severe hypotension. Interpret the ABG and identify what measures are probably indicated.

The PaO_2 of 38 mmHg tell us there is _____ hypoxemia. | *severe*

The patient is hyperventilating, as indicated by the low
_____. | *$PaCO_2$*

There is a large _____ gradient, indicating problems with gas exchange. | *A-aDO₂*

The very low blood pH indicates severe _____. | *acidemia*

The $PaCO_2$ is low, telling us the patient is hyperventilating and there is a respiratory _____. | *alkalosis*

The [HCO_3^-] of 9 mEq/L indicates the presence of a severe metabolic _____. | *acidosis*

The anion gap is _____ mEq/L. | *37*

In the presence of severe hypoxemia and hypotension, the increased anion gap metabolic acid-base disorder is probably due to _____ acidosis. | *lactic*

Note: In the setting of severe acidemia and cardiovascular compromise, treatment with HCO_3^- would be appropriate.

The initial dose of HCO_3^- to be given would be _____ mEq. | *210*

241

```
ABG No. 2
    pH = 7.49              Na⁺ = 141 mEq/L

PaCO₂ = 39 mmHg           Cl⁻ =  97 mEq/L

  PaO₂ = 66 mmHg

  HCO₃⁻ = 30 mEq/L
```

One hour after the patient was given HCO_3^-, ABG No. 2 and these electrolyte values were obtained. What is your interpretation now?

The PaO_2 now indicates a _____ hypoxemia.   *mild*

The patient's ventilatory status is now _____.   *normal*

The A-aDO₂ is now approximately _____ mmHg.   *35*

The patient's pH has become _____.   *alkalemic*

The $PaCO_2$ has gone from 25 to 39 and there is no longer any respiratory _____.   *alkalosis*

The [HCO_3^-] has risen from 9 to 30, indicating the onset of metabolic _____.   *alkalosis*

The anion gap is now within _____ range.   *normal*

Note: The house officer miscalculated and accidentally administered 420 mEq of HCO_3^-. At the same time, the patient's blood pressure improved with pressor agents and O_2 therapy and the lactic acidosis quickly resolved. The end result was iatrogenic-induced metabolic alkalemia.

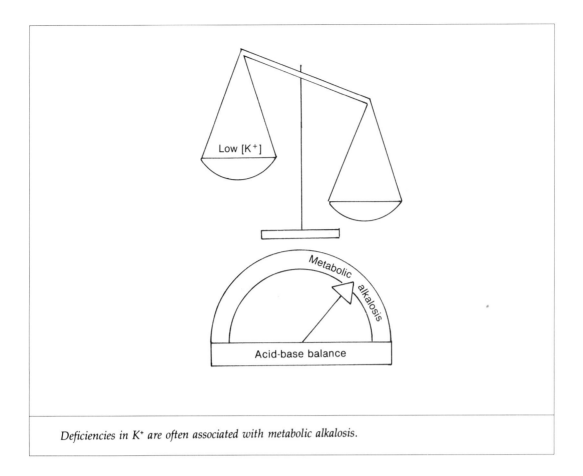

Deficiencies in K^+ are often associated with metabolic alkalosis.

Note: During metabolic alkalosis, H^+ will leave cells to help buffer the alkalosis. At the same time, K^+ will shift into the cells. The kidney also excretes more K^+ and conserves H^+. Consequently, metabolic alkalosis is usually associated with a fall in the serum K^+ (i.e., hypokalemia).

In metabolic alkalosis, the plasma K^+ is often _____.

low

Note: Severe K^+ losses can also cause a primary metabolic alkalosis. Since most K^+ is stored inside cells, K^+ deficits (e.g., as from poor dietary intake or excessive renal or gastrointestinal loss) will cause a shift of K^+ out of cells in an attempt to maintain the serum K^+ level within narrow limits. As K^+ leaves the cell, H^+ enters to maintain electrical balance inside the cell. This leads to a relative deficit of H^+ in the plasma, which will further aggravate metabolic alkalosis.

Severe K^+ losses can cause metabolic _____.

alkalosis

Metabolic alkalosis will cause a shift of K^+ into cells, leading to _____.

hypokalemia

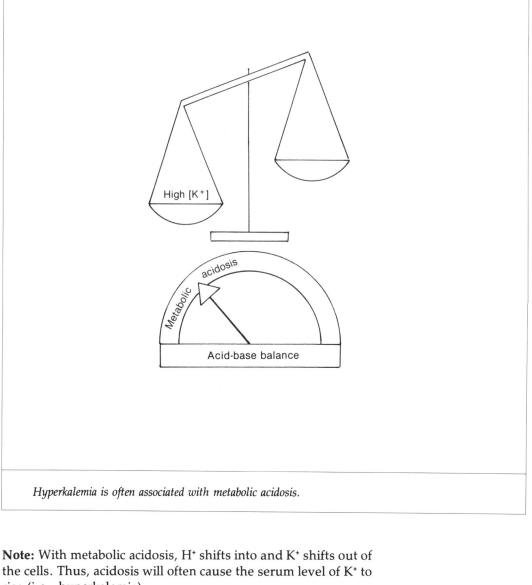

Hyperkalemia is often associated with metabolic acidosis.

Note: With metabolic acidosis, H^+ shifts into and K^+ shifts out of the cells. Thus, acidosis will often cause the serum level of K^+ to rise (i.e., hyperkalemia).

With metabolic acidosis, _____ leaves the cells and enters the blood.

K^+

Metabolic acidosis is often associated with a rise in serum K^+, or _____.

hyperkalemia

Note: There are several clinical situations in which metabolic acidosis may not be associated with hyperkalemia. In these cases, the primary disorders causing metabolic acidosis are often coupled with severe K^+ loss from the gastrointestinal or renal system (e.g., severe diarrhea or renal tubular acidosis).

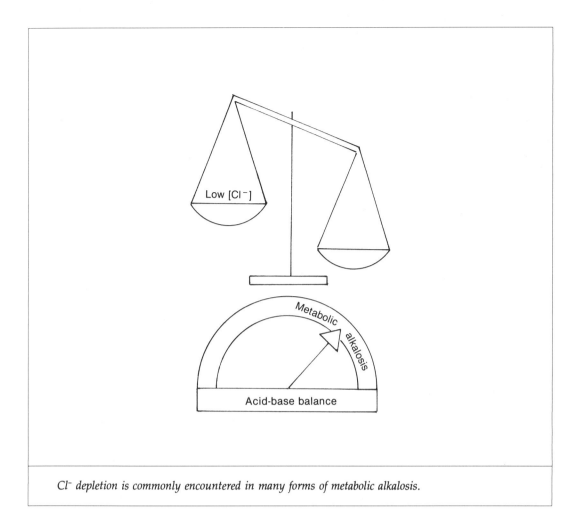

Cl⁻ depletion is commonly encountered in many forms of metabolic alkalosis.

Note: Cl^- and HCO_3^- are the largest contributors of negative charges to the blood. As the level of one decreases, the body will try to compensate by increasing the level of the other and vice versa.

As the blood Cl^- levels decrease, the HCO_3^- levels will _____ in the body's attempt to maintain electrical neutrality.

increase

Low plasma levels of Cl^- (hypochloremia) are common in metabolic _____.

alkalosis

Note: Some causes of metabolic acidosis are associated with hyperchloremia. These typically occur when there has been a primary loss of HCO_3^- resulting in an equivalent increase in serum Cl^- (normal anion gap acidosis).

Metabolic acidosis may sometimes be associated with _____.

hyperchloremia

Bibliography

Bea, M., and Thier, S. Mixed acid base disturbances: A clinical approach. *Med. Clin. North Am.*, 65 : 2, 1981.

Bear, R., and Gribik, M. Assessing acid-base imbalances through laboratory parameters. *Hosp. Pract.*, Nov., 1974.

Emmett, M., and Narins, R. Clinical use of the anion gap. *Medicine* 56 : 1, 1977.

Filley, G. Acid regulation and CO_2 retention. *Chest*, 58 (Suppl. 2), 1970.

Kaehny, W. Respiratory acid-base disorders. *Med. Clin. North Am.* 67 : 4, 1983.

McCurdy, D. Mixed metabolic and respiratory acid-base disturbances: Diagnosis and treatment. *Chest* 62 (Suppl. 2), 1972.

Narins, R., and Gardner, L. Simple acid-base disturbances. *Med. Clin. North Am.* 65 : 2, 1981.

Nawne, R., and Emmett, M. Simple and mixed acid-base disorders: A practical approach. *Medicine* 59 : 3, 1980.

Oh, M., and Carroll, H. The anion gap. *N. Engl. J. Med.* 297 : 15, 1977.

Simmons, D. Evaluation of acid-base status. *Basics of RD* 2 : 3, 1974.

Winters, R. W., and Dell, R. B. *Acid-Base Physiology in Medicine:* A Self-Instruction Program (3rd ed.). Boston: Little, Brown, 1982.

Table 5-1. Common causes of simple acid-base disorders

Metabolic acidosis	Metabolic alkalosis
Normal anion gap	
Primary HCO_3^- loss	Primary H^+ loss
From gastrointestinal tract	Persistent vomiting
Severe diarrhea	Nasogastric suction
Ileostomy	Diuretic prescription
Colostomy	Chronic steroid prescription
From kidneys	Exogenous HCO_3^-
Renal tubular acidosis	Severe K^+ depletion
Exogenous addition of acids containing Cl^-	
Ammonium chloride	
Hydrochloric acid	
Increased anion gap	
Exogenous addition of acids	
Salicylates	
Methanol	
Increased metabolic acid formation	
Diabetic keto acid	
Uremic acid	
Lactic acid	

Respiratory acidosis	Respiratory alkalosis
Acute or chronic lung disease	Lung disease
Severe chronic obstructive pulmonary diseases	Early restrictive disease
	Early obstructive disease
Acute airway obstruction	CNS disorders
CNS depression	Tumors
Drug overdose	Infection
Lesions of the respiratory control center	Anxiety
Neuromuscular disorders	Hypoxemia
Chest wall disorders	Gram-negative sepsis
Mechanical ventilator malfunction	Liver disease
	Ventilator induced

Table 5-2. Recognition of simple acid-base disorders

Disorder	pH	PaCO$_2$	HCO$_3^-$
Respiratory acidosis	↓	↑	↑* or N
Respiratory alkalosis	↑	↓	↓* or N
Metabolic acidosis	↓	↓* or N	↓
Metabolic alkalosis	↑	↑* or N	↑

*Present *if* physiologic compensation has taken place.
↓ = Decreased; ↑ = Increased; N = Normal.

Table 5-3. Expected compensation for simple acid-base disorders

Disorder	Initial change	Compensatory change	Expected degree of response
Metabolic acidosis	↓HCO$_3^-$	↓PaCO$_2$	Rapid decrease in PaCO$_2$ to bring pH approximately halfway back toward normal. Expected compensation quickly recognized by last two digits of PaCO$_2$ matching the last two digits of the pH.
Metabolic alkalosis	↑HCO$_3^-$	↑PaCO$_2$	Severe alkalemia *may* result in immediate PaCO$_2$ increase. PaCO$_2$ rarely rises over 50 mmHg. For every 1 mEq/L increase in [HCO$_3^-$] > 40 mEq/L, the PaCO$_2$ may increase by 1 mmHg.
Respiratory acidosis	↑PaCO$_2$	↑HCO$_3^-$	HCO$_3^-$ retention and H$^+$ excretion by kidneys begins immediately but takes several days for nearly complete compensation.
Respiratory alkalosis	↓PaCO$_2$	↓HCO$_3^-$	Kidney excretion of HCO$_3^-$ and retention of H$^+$ can often occur if condition persists for several days. Variable effectiveness, but compensation often results in at least partial return of pH toward normal.

↓ = Decreased; ↑ = Increased.

Table 5-4. Systematic approach to ABG interpretation

1. Assess PaO$_2$ to determine the oxygenation status.
2. Assess PaCO$_2$ to determine the ventilatory status.
3. Evaluate the A-aDO$_2$ to assess gas exchange.
4. Assess acid-base balance:
   a. Assess pH to determine the overall acid-base balance.
   b. Assess PaCO$_2$ and HCO$_3^-$ to determine the respiratory and metabolic status.
   c. Identify the primary acid-base disturbance (the pH will usually indicate which is primary).
   d. Evaluate the adequacy of compensation.
   e. Determine the nature of the acid-base disorder (acute or chronic? simple or mixed?).

6 Respiratory Failure

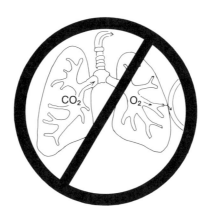

Many conditions may interfere with the primary functions of the respiratory system, which are to deliver O_2 to the blood and to remove CO_2.

One primary function of the respiratory system involves adequate delivery of _____ to the blood.

O_2

A second primary function of the respiratory system is to _____ CO_2 from the blood at the same rate that it is being added to the blood by cell metabolism.

remove

Note: By regulating the elimination of CO_2 from the body, the respiratory system also plays an important role in acid-base balance.

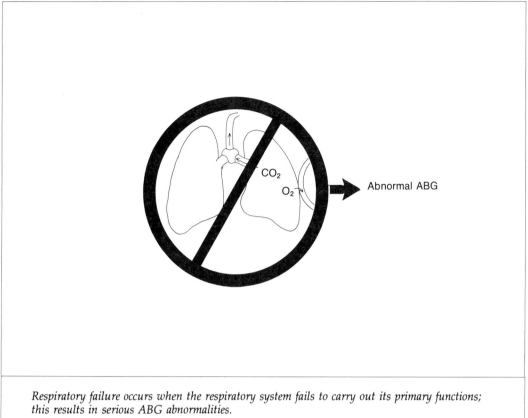

Respiratory failure occurs when the respiratory system fails to carry out its primary functions; this results in serious ABG abnormalities.

Failure of the _____ system results in serious ABG abnormalities.   *respiratory*

Serious blood-gas disturbances occur when the respiratory system _____ to carry out its primary functions.   *fails*

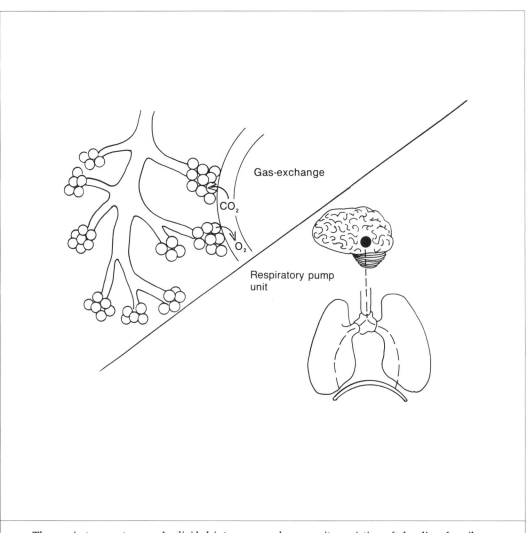

The respiratory system can be divided into a gas exchange unit consisting of alveoli and capillaries, and a respiratory pump unit consisting of the conducting airways and the respiratory muscles under central ventilatory control from the brainstem (medulla).

The gas-exchange unit consists of the _____ and _____.

alveoli
capillaries

Note: Remember, gas exchange occurs across the alveolar-capillary membrane and consists of O_2 diffusing from the alveoli into the blood and CO_2 diffusing out of the blood into the alveoli.

The respiratory pump unit consists of the airways and respiratory _____ under control from the brainstem.

muscles

The primary function of the respiratory pump is to generate alveolar ventilation to remove the _____ from the lungs.

CO_2

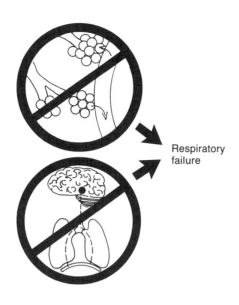

Respiratory failure

Respiratory failure can result from a breakdown in either the gas exchange unit or the respiratory pump unit of the respiratory system (or both).

Respiratory failure may develop from any condition that causes a breakdown in the _____ unit or the respiratory _____ unit.

gas exchange
pump

Note: There are hundreds of different conditions that can lead to respiratory failure. In practice, however, only a few are commonly encountered. Nevertheless, it is useful to realize the wide spectrum of diseases that are potential causes.

Although respiratory failure may be produced by many conditions, the end result is always a serious _____ abnormality.

ABG

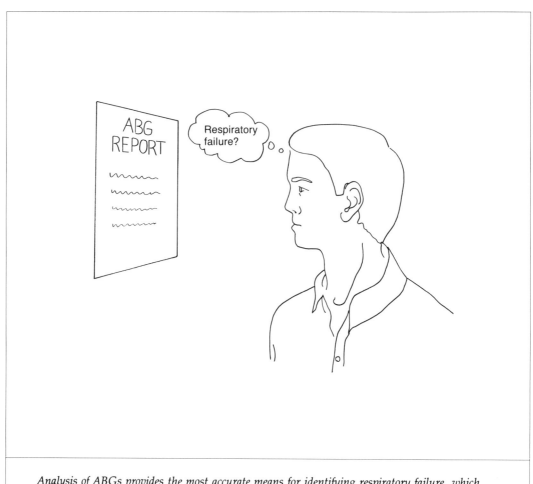

Analysis of ABGs provides the most accurate means for identifying respiratory failure, which often cannot be easily diagnosed on the basis of symptoms and physical findings alone.

Unless a patient is literally not breathing, respiratory failure is best diagnosed on the basis of _____ analysis.

ABG

Symptoms and physical findings alone are often _____ guides to the diagnosis of respiratory failure.

unreliable

The diagnosis of respiratory failure usually requires _____ puncture and measurements of PaO_2, $PaCO_2$, and pH.

arterial

```
        Respiratory failure ABGs
          pH ≈ normal/low
          PaO₂ ≈ low
          PaCO₂ ≈ normal/high
```

The typical ABG findings in respiratory failure are an abnormally low PaO₂, with or without a high PaCO₂, and a low pH.

In respiratory failure, the ABG will reveal an abnormally
_____ PaO$_2$.   *low*

The PaCO$_2$ may or may not be _____.   *elevated*

If the PaCO$_2$ is acutely elevated, the pH is usually _____. *low*

Note: There are no absolute levels of PaO$_2$, PaCO$_2$, and pH that define respiratory failure. The significance of these values in a particular patient depends on many factors such as clinical findings and prior blood-gas values for that patient. As a general guideline, a PaO$_2$ less than 60 mmHg or a PaCO$_2$ greater than 50 mmHg causing a pH less than 7.35 is used to indicate the presence of respiratory failure.

As you can see, there are several combinations of abnormal ABGs that can be classified as respiratory failure. For this reason, the diagnosis of respiratory failure by ABGs is usually divided into two types according to which of the two functions are most interfered with: *hypoxemic respiratory failure* (usually caused by defects in gas exchange) and *hypercapnic respiratory failure* (in which the primary problem usually involves the respiratory pump).

Respiratory failure

Hypoxemic	Hypercapnic
$\downarrow PaO_2$	$\uparrow PaCO_2$
	$\downarrow pH$

Based on the results of ABGs, two basic types of respiratory failure can be identified.

Respiratory failure can be divided into either _____ or _____ types according to the effect on ABGs.

hypoxemic
hypercapnic

Note: By classifying respiratory failure on the basis of ABGs into these two basic types, you will be able to understand how these differ in terms of pathogenesis, pathophysiology, clinical presentation, and therapy.

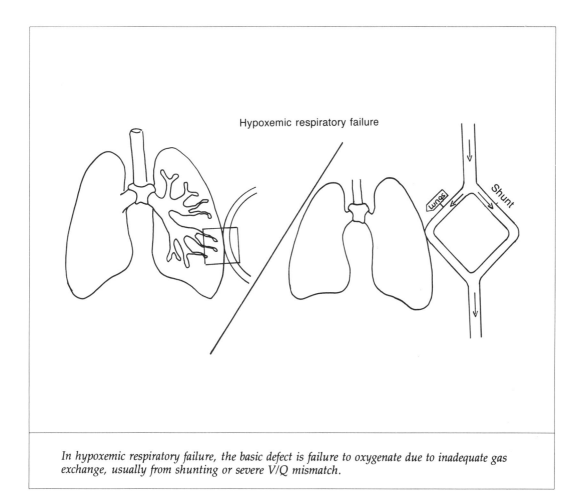

Hypoxemic respiratory failure

In hypoxemic respiratory failure, the basic defect is failure to oxygenate due to inadequate gas exchange, usually from shunting or severe V/Q mismatch.

_____ literally means low PaO_2 in the blood.   *Hypoxemia*

Hypoxemic respiratory failure refers to primary failure of the respiratory system to _____ arterial blood.   *oxygenate*

The inadequate gas exchange is usually from the two more common causes of hypoxemia: _____ or _____ mismatch.   *shunting, V/Q*

Note: Remember, there are other causes of hypoxemia including diffusion defects and decreased alveolar PO_2. However a diffusion defect is rarely severe enough to cause hypoxemic respiratory failure. Similarly, a decrease in the PAO_2 rarely causes the PaO_2 to fall to levels that lead to respiratory failure. If this were to occur, the primary problem would not be with the respiratory system, but rather with the quality of the air being breathed.

(At this time, a brief review of the causes of hypoxemia in Chap. 2, pp. 60–65 would probably be a good idea.)

```
┌─────────────────────────────────────────────────────────────────┐
│                                                                   │
│   Hypoxemic respiratory failure:                                  │
│                                                                   │
│   PaO₂ < 60 mmHg                                                  │
│                                                                   │
│                                                                   │
│                                                                   │
├───────────────────────────────────────────────────────────────────┤
│   Hypoxemic respiratory failure is characterized by a low PaO₂ (<60 mmHg). │
│                                                                   │
└─────────────────────────────────────────────────────────────────┘
```

A PaO_2 less than _____ usually constitutes _____ respiratory failure.   *60 mmHg, hypoxemic*

Note: Exactly when a low PaO_2 constitutes respiratory failure is, in part, arbitrary. We are really interested in the overall adequacy of the patient's oxygenation. Remember that at a PaO_2 of 60 mmHg, the saturation of Hb begins to fall rapidly. Hence, this is often considered the critical point for concern.

A PaO_2 less than 60 mmHg represents _____ hypoxemia.   *moderate*

Below a PaO_2 of 60 mmHg, the _____ of Hb begins to fall rapidly.   *saturation*

Note: Sometimes the PaO_2 may be less than 60 mmHg in the absence of respiratory failure. This situation can occur when there are anatomic right-to-left shunts (e.g., cardiac disease) or diminished O_2 tension in the environmental air (e.g., high altitude).

Hypoxemic respiratory failure
$PaO_2 \leqslant 60$ mmHg

+

$PaCO_2 \leqslant 40$ mmHg

In hypoxemic respiratory failure, alveolar ventilation is normal or increased so that the $PaCO_2$ is normal or reduced.

Respiratory failure associated with a low PaO_2 and a normal or low $PaCO_2$ is known as _____ respiratory failure.

hypoxemic

In hypoxemic respiratory failure, elimination of CO_2 is normal or _____.

increased

As a result, the _____ is normal or reduced.

$PaCO_2$

Note: Since hypoxemic respiratory failure primarily involves difficulties with gas exchange and not the respiratory pump (i.e., alveolar ventilation), there is usually no problem with elimination of CO_2. However, in the terminal stages of hypoxemic respiratory failure, CO_2 retention may occur as alveolar ventilation decreases and the $PaCO_2$ rises.

```
        Postoperative patient
                |
                v
        Hypoxemic respiratory failure          <------------- ARDS patient
                ^
                |
        Patient with severe pneumonia
```

Hypoxemic respiratory failure occurs in a wide variety of circumstances.

Note: One of the more common causes of hypoxemic respiratory failure is known as adult respiratory distress syndrome (ARDS). This causes massive shunting from atelectasis (i.e., collapsed alveoli) and edema in the lungs and results in the characteristic ABGs of hypoxemic failure. Synonyms include noncardiogenic pulmonary edema, shock lung, wet lung, leaky capillary syndrome, and diffuse pulmonary-capillary leak syndrome.

Hypoxemic respiratory failure can occur from _____ causes.

many

One of the more common causes is _____.

ARDS

Severe pneumonia in which many alveoli become filled with exudate can cause severe _____ and lead to hypoxemic respiratory failure.

shunting

A postoperative patient with atelectasis is at risk for developing _____ respiratory failure.

hypoxemic

$$pH = 7.48$$

$$PaCO_2 = 32 \text{ mmHg}$$

$$PaO_2 = 55 \text{ mmHg}$$

$$HCO_3^- = 24 \text{ mEq/L}$$

These blood gases were taken from a 35-year-old woman who complained of cough, fever, and shortness of breath. Based on the ABG results, what is your diagnosis?

A systematic review of the ABG reveals the following:

The PaO_2 indicates _____ hypoxemia.   *moderate*

The low _____ tells us the patient is hyperventilating.   *PaCO₂*

The low PaO_2 and the low $PaCO_2$ indicate there is a _____   *widened*
A-aDO₂ gradient.

The blood pH is high, indicating there is an _____.   *alkalemia*

Since the $PaCO_2$ is low, the patient has a respiratory _____.   *alkalosis*

The level of HCO_3^- tells us the patient's metabolic status is

_____.   *normal*

The high pH, the low $PaCO_2$, and the normal $[HCO_3^-]$ probably
indicate that we are dealing with an _____ respiratory   *acute*
alkalosis.

Since the PaO_2 is less than 60 mmHg and the $PaCO_2$ is low, our
ABG diagnosis is _____ respiratory failure.   *hypoxemic*

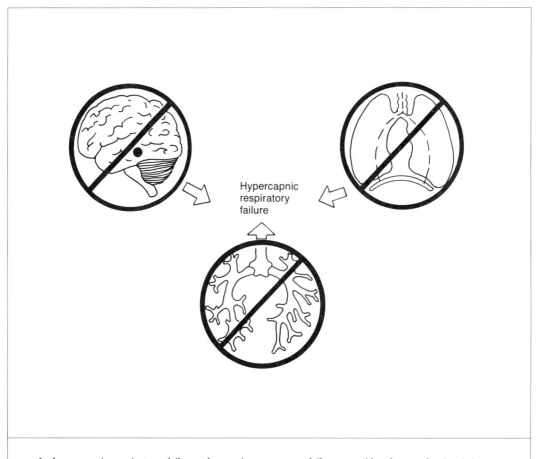

Hypercapnic
respiratory
failure

In hypercapnic respiratory failure, the respiratory pump fails to provide adequate levels of alveolar ventilation, causing the $PaCO_2$ to rise to dangerous levels.

Normally, there is a balance between metabolic production of _____ and its elimination by the respiratory system through the process of alveolar ventilation.

CO_2

Disorders that impair the ability of the respiratory system to remove CO_2 can lead to _____ respiratory failure.

hypercapnic

It is failure of the respiratory _____ that causes the inadequate alveolar ventilation.

pump

Note: Failure of the respiratory pump may result from a variety of pathologic processes affecting central ventilatory control mechanisms (e.g., narcotic overdose), respiratory neuromuscular function (e.g., myasthenia gravis), chest wall movement (e.g., flail chest), or any lung airway pathology so severe as to prevent adequate alveolar ventilation (e.g., severe chronic obstructive pulmonary diseases [COPD].

> Hypercapnic respiratory failure
>
> pH < 7.35
>
> $PaCO_2 > 50$ mmHg
>
> ---
>
> *Acute hypercapnia in which the $PaCO_2$ is greater than 50 mmHg and the pH is less than 7.35 is called* hypercapnic respiratory failure.

Note: If hypercapnia is chronic in nature, it will usually not be associated with severe acidemia (refer to Chap. 5, pp. 203–210 for a review of acute and chronic hypercapnia).

A $PaCO_2$ of greater than _____ associated with a pH less than _____ is referred to as hypercapnic respiratory failure.

50 mmHg
7.35

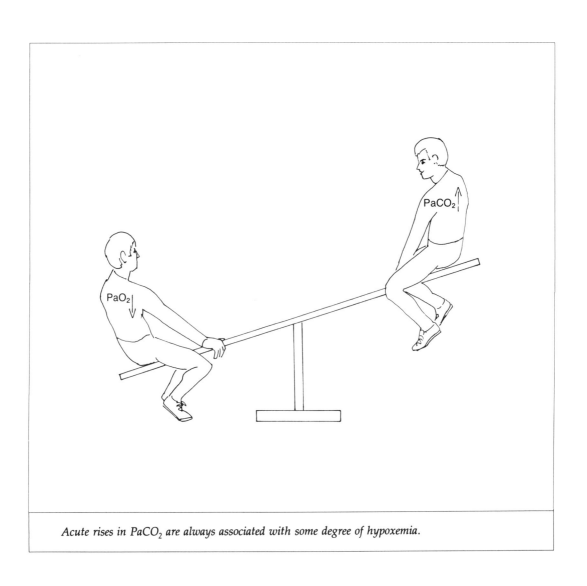

Acute rises in PaCO$_2$ are always associated with some degree of hypoxemia.

A rise in PaCO$_2$ is accompanied by a fall in _____ (assuming the patient is breathing room air).

PaO$_2$

The typical ABG abnormalities in hypercapnic respiratory failure are

PaCO$_2$ greater than _____

50 mmHg

pH less than _____ (indicating the acute status of the elevated PaCO$_2$)

7.35

PaO$_2$ less than _____ (at least until O$_2$ therapy is initiated)

normal

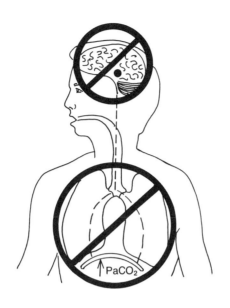

Hypercapnic respiratory failure may occur because of disorders of pulmonary or nonpulmonary origin, but it is always associated with failure of the respiratory pump resulting in CO_2 retention.

Hypercapnic respiratory failure may develop because of problems that are either pulmonary or _____ in origin.

nonpulmonary

Note: Knowledge of the types of disturbances contributing to hypercapnic respiratory failure is fundamental to diagnosis. (What part of the pump is failing? Is it a problem involving the chest wall, the ventilatory muscles, or the respiratory control center?) This assists in understanding the prognosis and providing successful management.

Hypercapnic respiratory failure is easily recognized on the basis of _____ analysis, but differentiation according to the site of the defect in the respiratory system is important.

ABG

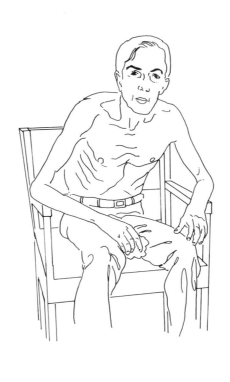

Hypercapnic respiratory failure most commonly occurs in patients with advanced COPD, most often emphysema and chronic bronchitis.

In most cases, hypercapnic respiratory failure develops in patients with underlying _____.

COPD

Emphysema and chronic _____ are conditions most commonly associated with hypercapnic respiratory failure.

bronchitis

Note: Patients with COPD often develop varying degrees of hypoxemia and hypercapnia. When these changes occur gradually, the body compensates by a variety of mechanisms (see Chap. 2, p. 70 and Chap. 5, pp. 202–208) and serious clinical disturbances may be prevented. These patients, although disabled by their disease, are nevertheless functionally stable from day to day. Respiratory failure develops when some further insult such as infection occurs causing worsening in gas exchange and failure of the respiratory pump. This is referred to as *acute respiratory failure superimposed on chronic respiratory insufficiency.*

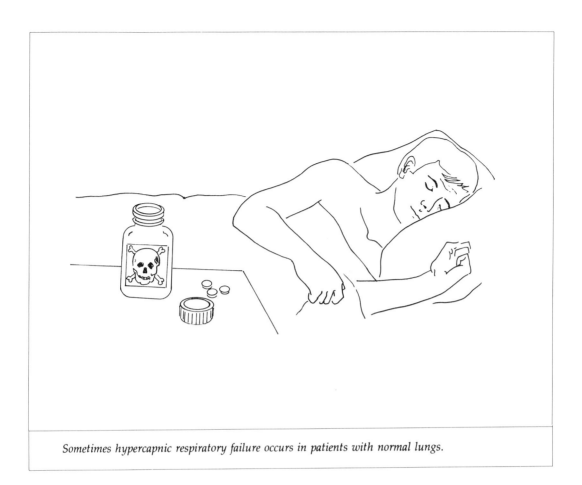

Sometimes hypercapnic respiratory failure occurs in patients with normal lungs.

On occasion, the respiratory pump fails to remove adequate amounts of CO_2 despite the presence of _____ lungs.

normal

In these situations, the primary disorder is of _____ origin.

nonpulmonary

Severe respiratory muscle _____ can cause acute hypercapnia.

fatigue

An excessive dose of sedatives could depress the respiratory _____ center and result in CO_2 retention.

control

↑ A-aDO$_2$ → Hypercapnic respiratory failure
(pulmonary origin)

Hypercapnic respiratory failure due to primary lung disorders is associated with disturbances in gas exchange as evidenced by widening of the A-aDO$_2$.

The _____ is a measure of the degree of gas exchange abnormality.

A-aDO$_2$

If the A-aDO$_2$ is greater than 12, this indicates the presence of a _____ abnormality.

gas exchange

Note: The larger the A-aDO$_2$, the more serious the gas exchange problem. (For a review of the calculation of A-aDO$_2$, see Chap. 4, pp. 121–123.)

```
┌─────────────────────────────────────────────────────────────┐
│                                                               │
│        Normal A-aDO₂ → Hypercapnic respiratory failure        │
│                    (non-pulmonary origin)                     │
│                                                               │
│                                                               │
├─────────────────────────────────────────────────────────────┤
│  A normal A-aDO₂ in association with hypercapnic respiratory   │
│  failure indicates that the primary disturbance is not of     │
│  lung origin.                                                 │
└─────────────────────────────────────────────────────────────┘
```

Causes of hypercapnic respiratory failure associated with normal _____ include disturbances in ventilatory drive, respiratory neuromuscular function, or chest-wall movement.

A-aDO₂ or gas exchange

Note: In reality, a combination of disturbances usually contributes to hypercapnic respiratory failure.

In a patient who overdoses on narcotics and develops respiratory center depression with an elevated $PaCO_2$, low PaO_2, but no increase in A-aDO₂, we would conclude that the lungs are exchanging gas _____.

normally

Even though a patient has hypercapnic respiratory failure, gas exchange may be _____.

normal

If a patient aspirates and develops pneumonia, one would expect a _____ of the A-aDO₂.

widening

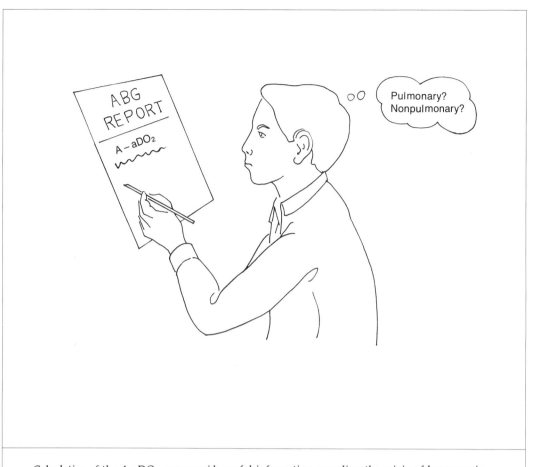

Calculation of the A-aDO₂ may provide useful information regarding the origin of hypercapnic respiratory failure.

When analyzing ABG results in hypercapnic respiratory failure, one should _____ the A-aDO$_2$.

calculate

Gas exchange problems often occur in hypercapnic respiratory failure and are recognized on the basis of the _____.

A-aDO$_2$

If the A-aDO$_2$ is increased, there are gas-exchange problems and the origin of the respiratory pump failure is, at least in part, due to primary _____ problems.

lung

If the A-aDO$_2$ is normal (< 12 mmHg on air), the cause of respiratory failure is _____ in origin (e.g., muscle, chest wall, or ventilatory control center problems).

nonpulmonary

Note: Calculation of the A-aDO$_2$ is also useful in evaluation of the degree of gas-exchange abnormality in hypoxemic respiratory failure.

$$pH = 7.20$$
$$PaCO_2 = 71 \text{ mmHg}$$
$$PaO_2 = 38 \text{ mmHg}$$
$$HCO_3^- = 26.5 \text{ mEq/L}$$

These blood gases were taken from a 16-year-old male who overdosed on narcotics. What is your ABG diagnosis? Is there any primary lung disease?

The PaO_2 of 38 mmHg indicates there is _____ hypoxemia.   *severe*

The $PaCO_2$ of 71 mmHg tells us the patient is _____.   *hypoventilating*

Since the $PaCO_2$ is 31 mmHg above an expected normal level of 40 mmHg, the PaO_2 would be expected to be reduced by approximately the _____ amount (see Chap. 2, p. 48).   *same*

Since the PaO_2 is decreased by more than 31, we know there is a _____ problem.   *gas exchange*

The gas-exchange abnormality is demonstrated by the increased _____.   *A-aDO$_2$*

The low blood pH indicates there is _____.   *acidemia*

The $PaCO_2$ is high, telling us there is a _____ acidosis.   *respiratory*

The HCO_3^- level indicates the metabolic acid-base status is _____.   *normal*

The low pH, high $PaCO_2$ and normal HCO_3^-, indicate we are probably dealing with an acute or _____ respiratory acidosis.   *uncompensated*

Since the $PaCO_2$ is 71 mmHg and the pH is 7.20, the ABG diagnosis is _____ respiratory failure.   *hypercapnic*

Note: A chest x ray confirmed the presence of an aspiration pneumonia. Remember that even when hypercapnic respiratory failure occurs on a primarily nonpulmonary basis (e.g., narcotic overdose), there are often superimposed lung problems.

Acute $\uparrow PaCO_2$ = Acidemia

In hypercapnic respiratory failure, acute retention of CO_2 leads to serious acid-base disturbances.

By removing CO_2 from the blood, the respiratory system plays an important role in acid-base _____.

balance

Respiratory disorders that lead to retention of _____ will cause changes in acid-base balance.

CO_2

In hypercapnic respiratory failure, serious acid-base disturbances are usually due to _____ retention of CO_2.

acute

The acute retention of CO_2 is recognized by _____.

acidemia

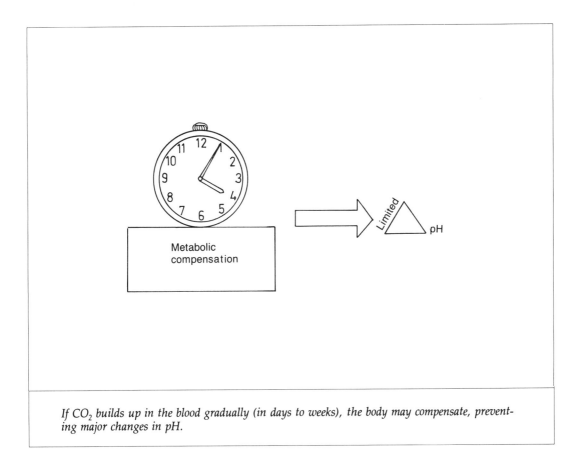

If CO_2 builds up in the blood gradually (in days to weeks), the body may compensate, preventing major changes in pH.

CO_2 may accumulate in the blood under certain conditions without major changes in _____.

pH

This occurs when the CO_2 builds up gradually and the body is able to _____.

compensate

In chronic CO_2 retention, blood pH is nearly _____.

normal

Note: If a patient has preexisting lung disease resulting in gradual retention of CO_2, compensatory metabolic changes tend to maintain a nearly normal pH despite the elevated $PaCO_2$. In these cases, *chronic respiratory insufficiency,* is sometimes misdiagnosed as acute respiratory failure.

$$pH = 7.39$$
$$PaCO_2 = 52 \text{ mmHg}$$
$$PaO_2 = 67 \text{ mmHg}$$
$$HCO_3^- = 31 \text{ mEq/L}$$

A patient with emphysema complained of chest tightness and went to a hospital emergency room where the above ABGs were obtained. What is your analysis?

The PaO_2 is 67 mmHg; there is only a _____ hypoxemia.   *mild*

The $PaCO_2$ indicates the patient is _____.   *hypoventilating*

The patient's A-aDO$_2$ is approximately _____ mmHg.   *18*

Note: This A-aDO$_2$ indicates only a mild gas exchange abnormality. The $PaCO_2$ rise of 12 mmHg above normal could account for part of the fall in PaO_2 but not for all of it.

The patient has a _____ pH.   *normal*

The $PaCO_2$ indicates a respiratory _____.   *acidosis*

The high [HCO_3^-] tells us there is a _____ alkalosis.   *metabolic*

The normal pH, high $PaCO_2$ and high HCO_3^-, indicate we are probably dealing with a _____ respiratory acidosis.   *chronic*

We could also call this chronic _____ or chronic _____.   *hypoventilation hypercapnia*

Note: This could also be called chronic respiratory insufficiency. Is it any wonder why this could be confusing? There are at least four ways of describing this ABG! Since this patient's respiratory and acid-base status seem stable, the chest tightness may be a result of heart disease.

$$pH = 7.31$$

$$PaCO_2 = 67 \text{ mmHg}$$

$$PaO_2 = 51 \text{ mmHg}$$

$$HCO_3^- = 33.5 \text{ mEq/L}$$

One week later, the same patient developed a cough and became more short of breath. The patient returned to the hospital where another ABG sample was obtained. What do you think?

The PaO_2 of 51 mmHg tells us there is a moderate degree of
_____ present.   *hypoxemia*

The increasing $PaCO_2$ indicates a worsening of the patient's
_____.   *hypoventilation*

The fall in PaO_2 in association with a rise in $PaCO_2$ indicates a
worsening of _____ exchange.   *gas*

The low blood pH indicates an _____.   *acidemia*

Since the pH is low and the $PaCO_2$ is high, there is a primary respiratory _____.   *acidosis*

The level of HCO_3^- indicates the presence of partial metabolic
_____ (i.e., compensatory metabolic alkalosis).   *compensation*

Knowing this patient's baseline ABGs enables us to make the
determination that this is an _____ respiratory acido-   *acute*
sis superimposed on chronic respiratory acidosis.

Note: Any reduction in arterial pH below 7.35 in an individual
with COPD and chronic CO_2 retention generally reflects acute
deterioration in ventilatory function and the onset of acute respiratory failure.

The patient now meets the ABG criteria for the diagnosis of
_____ respiratory failure.   *hypercapnic*

Note: Although the patient has developed acute hypercapnic respiratory failure, it is important to keep in mind the baseline
ABGs. The goal of therapy would be directed at returning this
patient to the baseline ABG values of PaO_2, $PaCO_2$ and pH,
rather than normal values.

Respiratory failure

Hypoxemic	Hypercapnic
$PaO_2 < 60$ mmHg	$PaO_2 <$ normal
$PaCO_2 < 40$ mmHg	$PaCO_2 > 50$ mmHg
	pH < 7.35

On the basis of ABGs, respiratory failure may be divided into two types: one in which there is a low PaO_2 but a normal or low $PaCO_2$, and the other in which the PaO_2 is also low but the $PaCO_2$ is high with a low pH.

Different types of respiratory _____ are associated with different degrees of hypoxemia and CO_2 retention.

failure

The only way to recognize the specific type of respiratory failure is on the basis of _____ analysis.

ABG

In _____ respiratory failure, the $PaCO_2$ can be normal or low.

hypoxemic

_____ respiratory failure is recognized by a $PaCO_2$ greater than 50 mmHg and a pH less than 7.35.

Hypercapnic

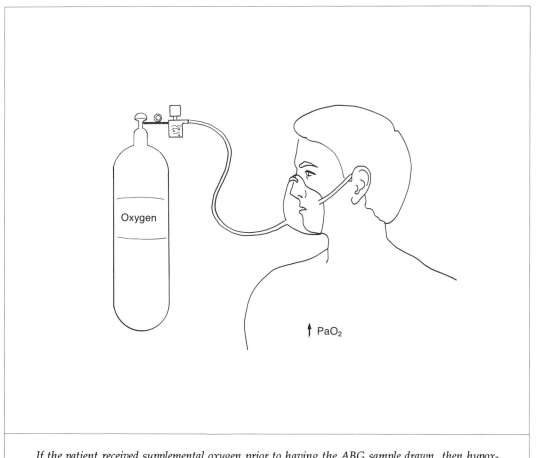

If the patient received supplemental oxygen prior to having the ABG sample drawn, then hypoxemia may have been abolished.

When ABG samples are drawn, the PaO$_2$ level will depend on the inspired concentration of _____.

O_2

In hypoxemic respiratory failure, arterial blood drawn from a patient breathing room air will show a PaO$_2$ less than _____.

60 mmHg

If a patient has received _____ O$_2$ beforehand, this may raise the PaO$_2$ and abolish hypoxemia.

supplemental

Note: Although hypoxemia may disappear following administration of O$_2$ therapy, there will still be an increased A-aDO$_2$ to indicate a gas exchange abnormality.

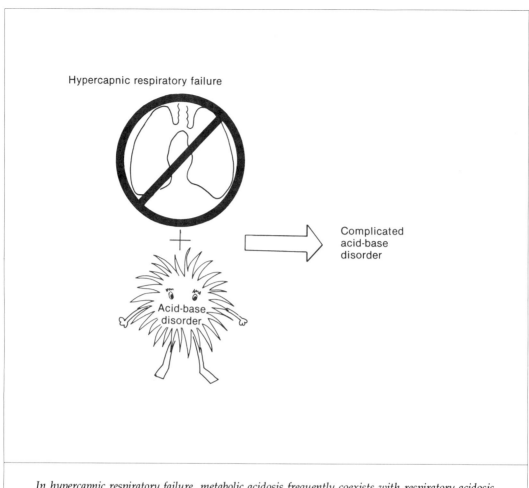

Hypercapnic respiratory failure

+

Acid-base disorder

Complicated acid-base disorder

In hypercapnic respiratory failure, metabolic acidosis frequently coexists with respiratory acidosis and complicates the acid-base disorder.

Note: In the setting of hypercapnic respiratory failure, metabolic acidosis is usually caused by the liberation of lactic acid from hypoxic tissues, which results from hypoxemia and circulatory disturbances.

Acidosis in respiratory failure can be of respiratory or _____ origin.

metabolic

In hypercapnic respiratory failure, acidosis is usually _____ in origin, but with tissue hypoxia, a metabolic component may also be detected.

respiratory

This combination is referred to as a _____ acidosis.

mixed or combined

The metabolic acidosis from tissue hypoxia comes from the production of _____ acid in the hypoxic cells.

lactic

$$pH = 7.18$$

$$PaCO_2 = 54 \text{ mmHg}$$

$$PaO_2 = 39 \text{ mmHg}$$

$$HCO_3^- = 19.5 \text{ mmHg}$$

A patient presents with the above ABG. What do you think?

The PaO_2 indicates _____ hypoxemia.   *severe*

Although the high $PaCO_2$ tells us the patient is _____,   *hypoventilating*
this cannot explain all of the decrease in the PaO_2.

There is an _____ A-aDO_2.   *increased*

The patient has a severe _____, as evidenced by the pH.   *acidemia*

The low pH in association with a high $PaCO_2$ and low $[HCO_3^-]$ indicates there is a combined respiratory and metabolic _____.   *acidosis*

The metabolic acidosis is probably due to tissue hypoxia resulting in _____ acid production.   *lactic*

Note: Immediate attention to correction of the hypoxemia and
acidemia is essential to this patient's survival.

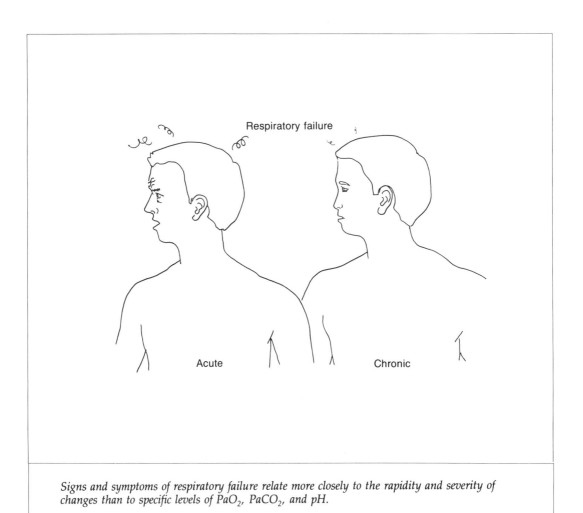

Signs and symptoms of respiratory failure relate more closely to the rapidity and severity of changes than to specific levels of PaO_2, $PaCO_2$, and pH.

Clinical findings in respiratory failure correlate more closely to *changes* than to _____ levels of PaO_2, $PaCO_2$, and pH.

specific

_____ disturbances in PaO_2, $PaCO_2$, and pH are poorly tolerated and clinical problems are usually obvious.

Acute

Patients who develop _____ abnormalities in blood gases tolerate significant degrees of hypoxemia and hypercapnia and may have minimal clinical findings.

gradual

ABG abnormalities of gradual onset are far less _____ than acute disturbances.

dangerous

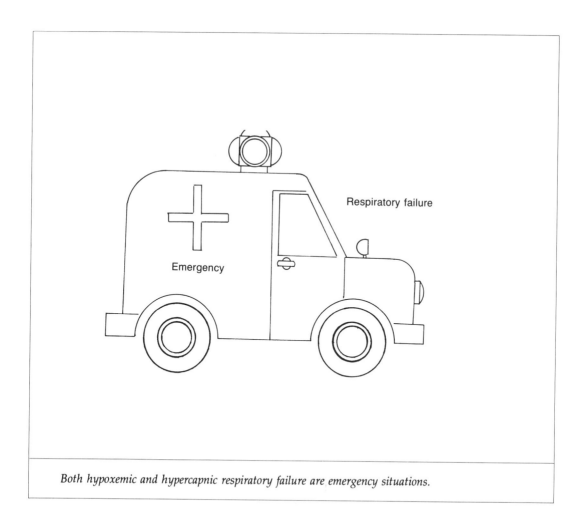

Both hypoxemic and hypercapnic respiratory failure are emergency situations.

Note: In hypercapnic respiratory failure, the rapid buildup of $PaCO_2$, fall in pH, and fall in PaO_2 in the blood have serious effects on cardiovascular and neurologic function. If left uncorrected for any prolonged period, death may ensue rapidly. Similarly, the low PaO_2 in hypoxemic respiratory failure is an immediate threat to life.

Respiratory failure is a medical _____ because it can rapidly cause death.

emergency

In respiratory failure, severe hypoxemia, hypercapnia, and acidemia must be treated _____ because they can pose a major threat to life.

immediately

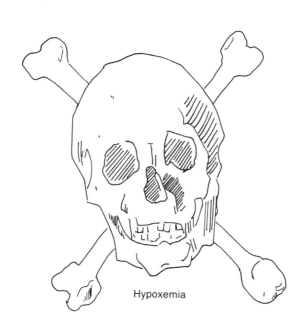

Hypoxemia

Hypoxemia is usually the most serious threat to patients with respiratory failure and must be promptly corrected.

_____, when severe enough, kills and does so quickly.

Hypoxemia

In all types of _____ failure, control of hypoxemia is of foremost importance.

respiratory

Note: Whereas low PaO_2 is dangerous, it is important to remember that PaO_2 is only one factor in the delivery of O_2 to the tissues. Other factors include the O_2 capacity of the blood, the O_2 affinity of the Hb, cardiac output, and distribution of blood flow.

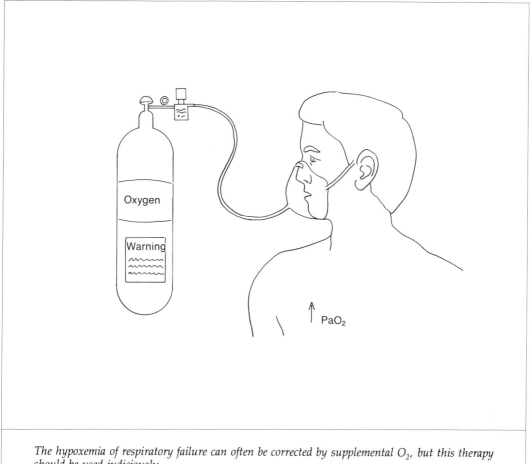

The hypoxemia of respiratory failure can often be corrected by supplemental O_2, but this therapy should be used judiciously.

In either type of respiratory failure, any reduction in PaO_2 below _____ usually requires treatment.

60 mmHg

Note: As a general rule, when the PaO_2 falls below 60 mmHg, O_2 therapy is recommended. At this level, the saturation of Hb begins to rapidly fall. However, O_2 should not be given unnecessarily. To review the hazards of O_2 therapy, see Chap. 2, pages 75–76.

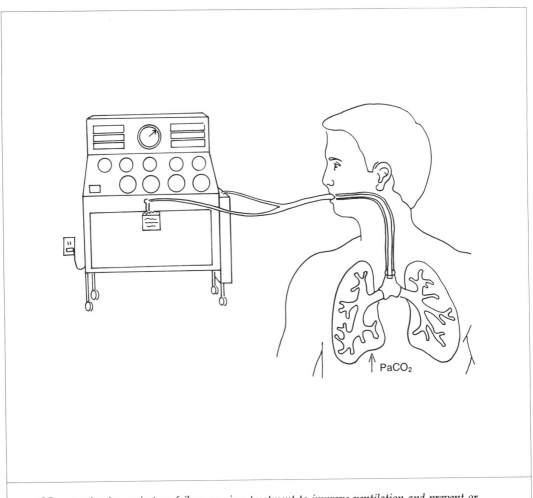

CO_2 retention in respiratory failure requires treatment to improve ventilation and prevent or eliminate excessive acidemia.

In hypercapnic respiratory failure, rapid rises in $PaCO_2$ reduce arterial pH and cause serious _____.

acidemia

Many of the detrimental effects of a high $PaCO_2$ are mediated through its effect on _____.

pH

Severe acidemia due to elevation of _____ must be corrected without delay and may require the use of mechanical ventilation.

$PaCO_2$

Note: It must be emphasized that the desired $PaCO_2$ is not always a normal $PaCO_2$. If the patient's baseline value of $PaCO_2$ is ordinarily high as a result of chronic disease it is desirable to mechanically ventilate only to that level of $PaCO_2$ when treating hypercapnic respiratory failure.

Patient with COPD on ventilator. ABG just prior to ventilator.

$$pH = 7.21$$
$$PaCO_2 = 88 \text{ mmHg}$$
$$PaO_2 = 46 \text{ mmHg}$$
$$HCO_3^- = 34.5 \text{ mEq/L}$$

ABG results from same patient 7 days later at discharge from hospital.

$$pH = 7.38$$
$$PaCO_2 = 53 \text{ mmHg}$$
$$PaO_2 = 62 \text{ mmHg}$$
$$HCO_3^- = 31 \text{ mEq/L}$$

The successful regulation of therapy in respiratory failure is best accomplished by serial analyses of ABGs.

Note: This patient has severe emphysema, developed pneumonia, and presented to the hospital with hypercapnic respiratory failure. His condition required the use of mechanical ventilation. After several days, his pneumonia cleared, mechanical ventilation was discontinued, and he returned to his previous baseline condition with the ABGs noted above. Note that this man is a chronic CO_2 retainer who had developed further CO_2 retention during his acute illness. His baseline level of $PaCO_2$ is not a normal level.

An interpretation of his baseline ABG is

The PaO_2 indicates a _____ hypoxemia.   *mild*

The $PaCO_2$ indicates the patient is _____ .   *hypoventilating*

The increased _____ indicates there is a gas-exchange abnormality.   *A-aDO₂*

Even though the pH is normal, the $PaCO_2$ and $[HCO_3^-]$ values suggest we are dealing with a primary _____ acidosis with a compensatory metabolic alkalosis.   *respiratory*

This acid-base picture is characteristic of _____ respiratory acidosis.   *chronic*

285

$$pH = 7.53$$

$$PaCO_2 = 43 \text{ mmHg}$$

$$PaO_2 = 86 \text{ mmHg}$$

$$HCO_3^- = 36 \text{ mEq/L}$$

The above ABG was obtained from a patient with severe COPD 1 hour after being intubated and placed on mechanical ventilation with 30 percent O_2. What is your ABG analysis?

While the patient's PaO_2 is normal, the patient is receiving 30 percent O_2. Therefore, the A-aDO_2 is _____.

increased

The high blood pH indicates an _____.

alkalemia

The _____ is normal. (Or is it?)

PaCO₂

The high [HCO_3^-] in association with a high pH suggests that the alkalemia is primarily _____ in origin.

metabolic

Note: This is the classic example of a chronic CO_2 retainer who has been overvigorously ventilated down to normal values. In this case, the patient had a chronic acidemia that was due to a primary respiratory acidosis (with a compensatory metabolic alkalosis). The overvigorous use of the ventilator had caused the patient to blow his $PaCO_2$ down to a level of 43 mmHg (from a usual $PaCO_2$ level in the 55-mmHg range) and produced another superimposed primary acid-base disturbance—namely a primary respiratory alkalosis. We would not be able to make this assessment without having the previous ABG values of this patient. Remember, the analysis phase of acid-base interpretation often necessitates the use of other data in addition to the single ABG in front of you (e.g., clinical data, prior ABGs).

$$pH = 7.34$$

$$PaCO_2 = 33 \text{ mmHg}$$

$$PaO_2 = 36 \text{ mmHg}$$

$$HCO_3^- = 18.4 \text{ mEq/L}$$

This is an ABG of a 33-year-old patient who presents with severe respiratory distress. The patient's chest x ray reveals pulmonary edema. What is your ABG interpretation and what do you think is the probable diagnosis?

The markedly reduced PaO_2 indicates the presence of severe
_____.   *hypoxemia*

The low $PaCO_2$ tells us the patient is _____.   *hyperventilating*

The A-aDO_2 is very large, indicating a severe _____   *gas exchange*
problem.

The low blood pH signifies the presence of _____.   *acidemia*

The combination of low pH, low $PaCo_2$ and low $[HCO_3^-]$ tells us
there is a respiratory _____ that appears to be com-   *alkalosis*
pensating for a primary _____ acidosis.   *metabolic*

Based on the PaO_2 and $PaCO_2$ values, our ABG diagnosis is
_____ respiratory failure.   *hypoxemic*

Note: Defining the type of respiratory failure is important because the treatment of the two types of failure differs. In this
case, the patient's hypoxemic respiratory failure was determined to be due to ARDS.

$$pH = 7.32$$
$$PaCO_2 = 78 \text{ mmHg}$$
$$PaO_2 = 50 \text{ mmHg}$$
$$HCO_3^- = 39.3 \text{ mEq/L}$$

What is your ABG analysis?

The PaO_2 values indicate a _____ degree of hypoxemia.

moderate

Note: Since the $PaCO_2$ is 38 mmHg above normal and the PaO_2 is about the same amount below normal, there does not appear to be a gas exchange problem. The fall in PaO_2 can be explained by the rise in $PaCO_2$.

The calculated A-aDO$_2$ is _____.

normal

The low blood pH indicates a mild _____.

acidemia

Since the $PaCO_2$ is high, this tells us there is a respiratory _____.

acidosis

In the setting of a low pH and high $PaCO_2$, the high [HCO_3^-] probably represents partial _____ compensation for the respiratory acidosis.

metabolic

On the basis of the PaO_2 of 50 mmHg, $PaCO_2$ of 78 mmHg, and pH of 7.32, our ABG diagnosis is _____ respiratory failure.

hypercapnic

Note: Whereas the ABG values indicate hypercapnic respiratory failure, the normal A-aDO$_2$ indicates the patient is able to exchange gas normally in the lungs. This situation might occur in acute drug overdose or other disorders in which the primary disturbance in ventilation is nonpulmonary in origin.

See Table 6-1 on page 294 for a review of formulas that are commonly used in ABG interpretation.

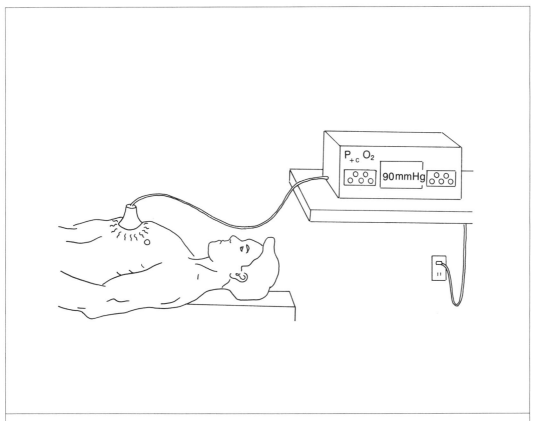

Although we usually rely on direct sampling of arterial blood to measure PaO_2, there are other noninvasive techniques available such as transcutaneous O_2 monitoring to help evaluate oxygenation.

Note: A heated probe placed on the skin causes vasodilation and a great increase in blood flow to that area of skin. Due to this high rate of perfusion, the PO_2 of capillary blood will approximate that of arterial blood. By monitoring O_2 diffusing through the skin, a specialized O_2 electrode can measure a patient's transcutaneous PO_2 ($P_{tc}O_2$).

O_2 in the capillaries perfusing the skin can be measured by a
_____ gas monitor.

transcutaneous

The PO_2 measured by this type of skin probe is referred to as the
_____.

$P_{tc}O_2$

Note: $P_{tc}O_2$ measurements primarily reflect the efficiency of O_2 delivery to the skin and may not necessarily be equal to the PaO_2. However, this technique can reveal changes in gas tensions and is a particularly popular method to monitor infants, for whom the expense and complications of frequent ABG monitoring can be minimized.

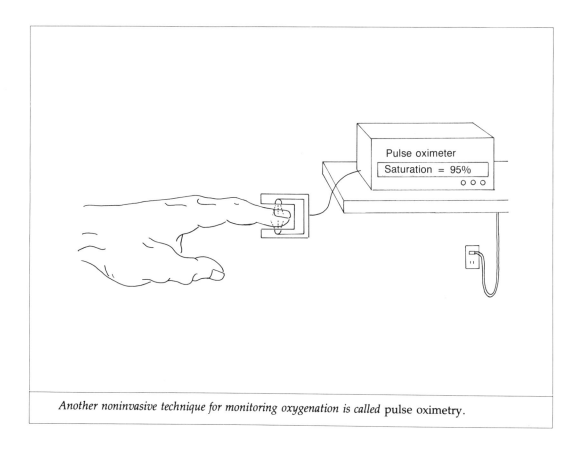

Another noninvasive technique for monitoring oxygenation is called pulse oximetry.

Note: Pulse oximetry is accomplished by measuring light transmission through a finger or ear. As a light passes through the arterial blood in the finger or earlobe, some of it is absorbed by oxygenated Hb. This level of light absorbance can be used to determine the O_2 saturation of the $Hb(SaO_2)$. A major advantage of oximetry is that changes in SaO_2 can be continuously monitored.

The oximetry technique involves measurement of _____ transmission through the ear or finger and its absorption by oxygenated Hb.

light

Oximetry readings closely approximate the directly measured _____.

SaO_2

Note: Although oximetry is usually considered accurate within ± 1 percent, the presence of unusual types of Hb (e.g., carboxyhemoglobin) can result in erroneous measurements.

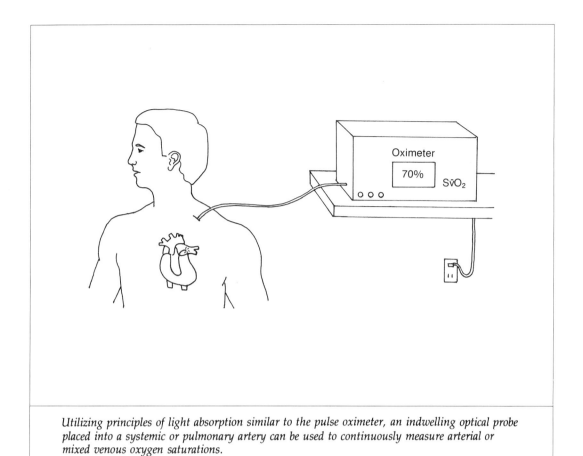

Utilizing principles of light absorption similar to the pulse oximeter, an indwelling optical probe placed into a systemic or pulmonary artery can be used to continuously measure arterial or mixed venous oxygen saturations.

The O_2 saturation of arterial blood can be measured on a _____ basis with the use of a special catheter.

continuous

Measurements of mixed venous oxygenation made by a pulmonary artery catheter can be used to assess _____ oxygenation.

tissue

Note: The primary disadvantage of this type of monitoring is the added risk of complications associated with placement of indwelling catheters (e.g., infection, ischemia, thrombus formation). As with pulse oximetry, significant levels of carboxyhemoglobin or methemoglobin can result in erroneous readings. If either of these conditions is suspected, another type of measurement capable of detecting these abnormal hemoglobins should be performed (i.e., cooximetry).

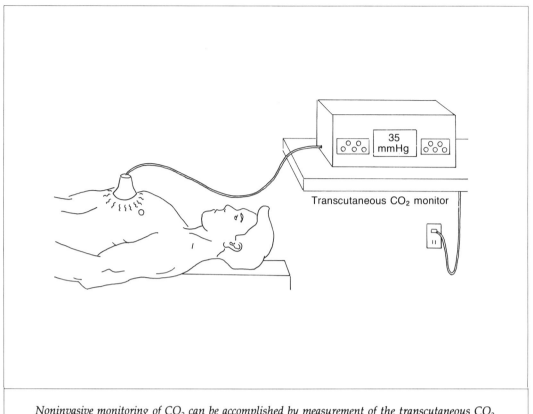

Noninvasive monitoring of CO_2 can be accomplished by measurement of the transcutaneous CO_2 gas tension ($P_{tc}CO_2$).

Note: Both the $P_{tc}O_2$ and the $P_{tc}CO_2$ can be measured from a single skin probe. In a technique similar to the $P_{tc}O_2$ measurement, the level of CO_2 in the capillary blood can be estimated by a skin probe. Although this technique does not measure actual levels of $PaCO_2$, it can be used to monitor for relative changes in ventilation. Trends of increasing or decreasing $P_{tc}CO_2$ are, however, best validated by direct ABG measurements.

Using noninvasive techniques, continuous measurements of $P_{tc}CO_2$ can be used to monitor for relative changes in _____.

ventilation or PaCO$_2$

A trend of increasing $P_{tc}CO_2$ indicates the need for an _____ to be performed.

ABG

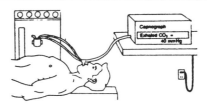

Another noninvasive method of monitoring CO_2 is analysis of exhaled gas. This technique is referred to as capnography.

Note: Under most circumstances, there is very little difference between the alveolar and arterial PCO_2 ($P\text{A}CO_2 \approx PaCO_2$). Based on this concept, exhaled air can be analyzed for PCO_2, with the measurement obtained during the last portion of the exhalation (*end-tidal* CO_2) being used to approximate the $P\text{A}CO_2$. This provides a close estimate of the $PaCO_2$. An estimation of the arterial PCO_2 from measurements of the alveolar PCO_2 is acceptable for many clinical purposes. However, in patients with severe lung diseases and abnormalities in the distribution of ventilation, there are marked limitations to this technique and supplemental measurements of ABGs are necessary to validate results.

Analysis of exhaled gas for CO_2 is referred to as _____.

capnography

End-tidal PCO_2 measurements usually correlate with $P\text{A}CO_2$ and can provide a close estimate of the _____.

PaCO₂

Noninvasive techniques for measuring PCO_2 make no assessment of arterial pH and therefore cannot replace _____ determinations in acutely ill patients.

ABG

Bibliography

Burki, N., and Albert, R. Noninvasive monitoring of arterial blood gases. *Chest* 83 : 4, 1983.

Burrows, B., Knudson, R., and Kettel, L. *Respiratory Insufficiency.* Chicago: Year Book, 1975.

Guenter, C. A., and Welch, M. H. (eds.) *Pulmonary Medicine.* (2nd ed.). Philadelphia: Lippincott, 1982.

Martin, L. Respiratory failure. *Med. Clin. North Am.* 61 : 6, 1977.

Saunders, N., Prowles, A., and Rebuck, A. Ear oximetry: Accuracy and practicability in the assessment of arterial oxygenation. *Am. Rev. Respir. Dis.* 113, 1976.

Shapiro, B. A., Harrison, R. A., and Walton, J. R. *Clinical Application of Blood Gases* (3rd ed.). Chicago: Year Book, 1982.

West, J. B. *Pulmonary Pathophysiology: the Essentials* (2nd ed.), Baltimore: Williams & Wilkins, 1981.

Table 6-1. Formulas commonly used in ABG interpretation

Name	Formula	Information provided
Alveolar air equation	$P_AO_2 = (P_{atm} - PH_2O) \times FIO_2 - PaCO_2/R$	Estimate of average alveolar oxygen tension
Alveolar-arterial oxygen gradient	$A\text{-}aDO_2 = [(713 \times FIO_2) - (1.25 \times PaCO_2)] - PaO_2$	Estimate of degree of gas-exchange abnormality
Anion gap	$AG = [Na^+] - ([HCO_3^-] + [Cl^-])$	Assists with determination of etiology of metabolic acidosis
Carbonic acid concentration	$[H_2CO_3] = (0.03) \times PaCO_2$	Actual blood carbonic acid level
Correction of metabolic acidosis	HCO_3^- dose = [body wt (kg) $\times$ 0.40] $\times$ [24 $-$ actual HCO_3^-]	Dosage of HCO_3^- to correct deficit. Usually half this amount is given and then the ABGs are rechecked
Hydrogen ion concentration	$[H^+] = 24 \times PaCO_2/[HCO_3^-]$	Actual $[H^+]$ in nanomoles/L
Minute alveolar ventilation	$\dot{V}A = (V_T - V_D) \times f$	Alveolar ventilation is inversely related to the $PaCO_2$
Minute ventilation	$\dot{V}E = V_T \times f$	Total ventilation breathed in 1 minute
Oxygen content formula	$CaO_2 = (0.003) \times (PaO_2) + (1.36) \times (Hb) \times (SaO_2)$	Total oxygen content of the arterial blood in cc/dl of blood
Predicted PaO_2 with age	$PaO_2 = 80 -$ (number of years over 70)	Predicts normal decline in PaO_2 with aging

Appendix A   *Practice Problems*

$$pH = 7.33$$

$$PaCO_2 = 35 \text{ mmHg}$$

$$PaO_2 = 74 \text{ mmHg}$$

$$HCO_3^- = 18 \text{ mEq/L}$$

$$BE = -7.0$$

$$SaO_2 = 93.8\%$$

Baby D is a 4-hour-old premature infant who was placed in an oxygen hood with 25 percent O_2 due to respiratory distress and cyanosis immediately after birth. The first ABG reveals the above data. What is your interpretation?

Although the patient's PaO_2 is adequate, it does indicate a _____ hypoxemia.

mild

At this young age, the infant is still able to generate the massive inspiratory effort necessary to expand stiff lungs and is still able to _____ , as evidenced by the low $PaCO_2$.

hyperventilate

The A-aDO_2 is mildly _____ , indicating a gas exchange problem.

elevated

The pH indicates an _____ .

acidemia

There is a slight respiratory _____ and a metabolic _____ .

alkalosis
acidosis

This appears to be a _____ metabolic acidosis.

compensated

Note: Premature infants who have respiratory distress from birth are often diagnosed later as having respiratory distress syndrome (RDS). They often progressively deteriorate over the next 24 to 36 hours, when the disease reaches its peak.

$$pH = 7.25$$
$$PaCO_2 = 48 \text{ mmHg}$$
$$PaO_2 = 56 \text{ mmHg}$$
$$HCO_3^- = 20.6 \text{ mEq/L}$$
$$BE = -6.5$$
$$SaO_2 = 83.4\%$$

Baby D is now 18 hours old and is breathing 45 percent O_2 via an oxygen hood. There is evidence of increased distress (i.e., increased intercostal and sternal retractions and more tachypnea). Interpret the most recent ABG.

The PaO_2 demonstrates _____ hypoxemia.   *moderate*

The patient is _____, as seen by the low $PaCO_2$.   *hypoventilating*

The A-aDO_2 is _____ mmHg, indicating serious problems with gas exchange.   *169*

The low pH indicates _____.   *acidemia*

There is respiratory _____, as evidenced by the elevated $PaCO_2$.   *acidosis*

The _____ HCO_3^- indicates the presence of metabolic acidosis.   *low*

The low pH, high $PaCO_2$, and low HCO_3^- tell us we are dealing with a _____ metabolic and respiratory acidemia.   *mixed*

Note: This is a typical ABG of a premature infant who has RDS and is "fatigued." The massive shunt caused from collapse of unstable alveoli and excessive work of breathing lead to life-threatening degrees of hypoxemia, hypercapnia, and acidemia, often necessitating ventilatory support.

$$pH = 7.59$$

$$PaCO_2 = 20 \text{ mmHg}$$

$$PaO_2 = 53 \text{ mmHg}$$

$$HCO_3^- = 19.4 \text{ mEq/L}$$

$$BE = 0$$

$$SaO_2 = 92.8\%$$

A patient with the above ABG data was found unconscious in an abandoned building and brought to the emergency room where he had a respiratory arrest. He was resuscitated and placed on ventilatory support with an FIO$_2$ of 0.6. What is your ABG interpretation?

Despite supplemental O_2, the low PaO_2 indicates moderate
_____.

hypoxemia

The $PaCO_2$ of 20 mmHg tells us that the patient is being mechanically _____.

hyperventilated

This patient on an FIO$_2$ of 0.6 has an A-aDO$_2$ of _____ mmHg.

350

This widened A-aDO$_2$ indicates marked problems with _____ exchange.

gas

The pH indicates severe _____.

alkalemia

The low $PaCO_2$ indicates the presence of respiratory _____.

alkalosis

Note: Although the HCO_3^- is low, remember the effect a low $PaCO_2$ has on the HCO_3^-. An acute decrease of 20 mmHg will lower the HCO_3^- approximately 3 mEq/L. Hence, evaluating this HCO_3^- for the metabolic status would result in the determination that it is normal.

The high pH, low $PaCO_2$, and normal HCO_3^-, indicate that we are dealing with a primary or simple _____ alkalemia.

respiratory

Note: The cause of the respiratory alkalemia is clearly overzealous mechanical ventilation. Patients placed on ventilators are commonly overventilated in an attempt to normalize the $PaCO_2$. Unfortunately, overvigorous ventilation can have dangerous neurologic, cardiovascular, and acid-base consequences.

$$pH = 7.47$$
$$PaCO_2 = 34 \text{ mmHg}$$
$$PaO_2 = 75 \text{ mmHg}$$
$$HCO_3^- = 24.5 \text{ mEq/L}$$
$$BE = +2.0$$
$$SaO_2 = 95.9\%$$

The above ABG was obtained from a 14-year-old known asthmatic girl who presented to the emergency room with respiratory distress that developed over the past 2 hours. What is your interpretation of the ABG?

The PaO_2 of 75 mmHg indicates _____ hypoxemia.	*mild*
The $PaCO_2$ indicates slight _____.	*hyperventilation*
The A-aDO$_2$ is _____ mmHg.	*32*
The high pH indicates slight _____.	*alkalemia*
The $PaCO_2$ is low, indicating respiratory _____.	*alkalosis*
The metabolic status is _____.	*normal*
This appears to be an uncompensated _____ alkalosis.	*respiratory*

Note: This ABG is typical of those seen in mild to moderate asthma. If the asthmatic attack becomes severe, the patient will become more hypoxemic and, as fatigue sets in, the $PaCO_2$ will begin to climb. Life-threatening asthma is characterized by CO_2 retention, acidemia, and hypercapnic respiratory failure.

$$pH = 7.26$$

$$PaCO_2 = 29 \text{ mmHg}$$

$$PaO_2 = 107 \text{ mmHg}$$

$$HCO_3^- = 12 \text{ mEq/L}$$

$$BE = -13$$

$$SaO_2 = 97\%$$

$$Na^+ = 139 \text{ mEq/L}$$

$$Cl^- = 104 \text{ mEq/L}$$

Forty-two-year-old James Sweet came to the emergency room complaining of shortness of breath and had rapid and deep respirations. The above ABG and laboratory results were obtained. What is your ABG interpretation?

The PaO_2 of 107 mmHg on room air tells us that arterial oxygenation is _____.   *adequate*

The $PaCO_2$ of 29 mmHg means the patient is _____.   *hyperventilating*

The A-aDO_2 of 7 indicates that gas exchange is _____.   *normal*

The low pH of 7.26 indicates a severe degree of _____.   *acidemia*

There is a respiratory alkalosis as evidenced by the low $PaCO_2$, and this is probably a _____ response.   *compensatory*

The low HCO_3^- and low pH tell us we are dealing with a primary _____ acidemia.   *metabolic*

By calculating the anion gap, we find it is _____ mEq/L.   *23*

We are dealing with an _____ anion gap metabolic acidosis.   *increased*

Note: The patient turned out to be an insulin-dependent diabetic who had gone into a diabetic crisis with a ketoacidosis. The additional load of keto acids caused the increase anion gap acidosis.

300

$$pH = 7.22$$

$$PaCO_2 = 84 \text{ mmHg}$$

$$PaO_2 = 39 \text{ mmHg}$$

$$HCO_3^- = 34.8 \text{ mEq/L}$$

$$BE = +0.5$$

$$SaO_2 = 62\%$$

Stella Speed was found in her apartment by neighbors. She was brought into the emergency room by paramedics, where the above ABG was obtained. What is your interpretation?

The PaO_2 of 39 mmHg indicates _____ hypoxemia.   *severe*

The $PaCO_2$ of 84 mmHg tells us there is marked _____.   *hypoventilation*

The A-aDO$_2$ value of _____ mmHg indicates no problem with gas exchange.   *6*

The pH indicates severe _____.   *acidemia*

Since the low pH is associated with a marked increase in $PaCO_2$, we are dealing with a primary _____ acidosis.   *respiratory*

The HCO_3^- of 34.8 probably indicates metabolic _____.   *compensation*

The low pH, markedly elevated $PaCO_2$, and low PaO_2 are diagnostic of _____ respiratory failure.   *hypercapnic*

Note: This type of ABG pattern is typical of hypercapnic respiratory failure, in which a low PaO_2 is associated with acute CO_2 retention and acidemia. The normal A-aDO$_2$ suggests that the primary problem is not of lung origin and is most likely secondary to a problem with the respiratory pump (see p. 262–265). In this case, the patient was a victim of an acute narcotic overdose.

$$pH = 7.43$$

$$PaCO_2 = 36 \text{ mmHg}$$

$$PaO_2 = 69 \text{ mmHg}$$

$$HCO_3^- = 24 \text{ mEq/L}$$

$$BE = 0$$

$$SaO_2 = 94.1\%$$

Thomas Puffer came to the hospital complaining of increasing difficulty in performing his daily activities. He found that he was "huffing and puffing" with even the slightest exertion. He appeared thin with pursed-lip breathing and a barrel-shaped chest. What is your ABG interpretation?

The PaO_2 of 69 mmHg denotes a _____ degree of hypoxemia.   *mild*

Ventilation is _____, as seen by the low $PaCO_2$.   *increased*

The A-aDO_2 is _____, telling us that gas exchange is impaired.   *widened*

The pH is slightly _____.   *alkaline*

The pH, $PaCO_2$, and HCO_3^- values tell us we are probably dealing with a primary _____ alkalemia.   *respiratory*

Note: This ABG pattern is typical of a "pink puffer." This term has been used to describe individuals with COPD (usually emphysema) who are able to maintain adequate levels of arterial oxygenation and alveolar ventilation (i.e., normal or low $PaCO_2$) despite their lung disease and increased work of breathing. As the disease progresses, these individuals may develop advancing degrees of hypoxemia, hypercapnia (hypoventilation), and acidemia.

$$pH = 7.39$$

$$PaCO_2 = 52 \text{ mmHg}$$

$$PaO_2 = 58 \text{ mmHg}$$

$$HCO_3^- = 33 \text{ mEq/L}$$

$$BE = +5.0$$

$$SaO_2 = 89.3\%$$

Martin Spitz is being seen in the clinic for a followup visit from a recent hospitalization. He is using O_2 via a nasal cannula at a rate of 1 L/min when the above ABG was obtained. What is your interpretation?

The PaO_2 of 58 mmHg indicates a _____ degree of hypoxemia.   *moderate*

The $PaCO_2$ of 52 mmHg tells us that Mr. Spitz is _____.   *hypoventilating*

There is a gas exchange abnormality, as evidenced by the presence of an increased _____.   *A-aDO$_2$*

Note: Even if Mr. Spitz were breathing room air, calculation of the A-aDO$_2$ tells us there is an increased gradient. We know that the patient is breathing 1 L/min of O_2 resulting in a further increase in the A-aDO$_2$.

Despite a _____ pH, the $PaCO_2$ is high indicating the   *normal*
presence of respiratory _____.   *acidosis*

The HCO_3^- is elevated, telling us there is also metabolic
_____.   *alkalosis*

This appears to be chronic _____ acidosis.   *respiratory*

Note: The high $PaCO_2$ and high HCO_3^- tell us we are dealing with a combination of respiratory acidosis and metabolic alkalosis. However, despite the presence of these acid-base changes, the overall pH is normal. Ordinarily, a single primary acid-base disorder is rarely fully compensated so that the final pH will deviate in the direction of the primary disorder. However, in this case, we are probably dealing with a primary respiratory acidosis that has been present for enough time to allow complete compensation (i.e., chronic respiratory acidosis).

$$pH = 7.35$$
$$PaCO_2 = 63 \text{ mmHg}$$
$$PaO_2 = 88 \text{ mmHg}$$
$$HCO_3^- = 34.5 \text{ mEq/L}$$
$$BE = +6.5$$
$$SaO_2 = 96\%$$

While Mr. Spitz was in the clinic for his appointment, it was discovered that the flow of O_2 had mistakenly been increased to 3 L/min. The above ABG was obtained on this O_2 flow. What is your interpretation?

The PaO_2 of 88 mmHg tells us that _____ has been abolished.

hypoxemia

The $PaCO_2$ has risen to 63 mmHg, indicating an increased degree of _____.

hypoventilation

The pH has dropped and become more _____.

acidic

In light of the rising $PaCO_2$, the increased degree of acidemia is _____ in origin.

respiratory

Note: Patients who chronically retain CO_2 are usually quite dependent on a hypoxic stimulus to breathe. If hypoxemia is abolished, they will lose their "hypoxic drive" to breathe and this will result in further depression of their ventilation and a worsening of respiratory acidosis. One must always be cautious when giving supplemental O_2 to patients who are chronic CO_2 retainers.

$$pH = 7.28$$
$$PaCO_2 = 69 \text{ mmHg}$$
$$PaO_2 = 49 \text{ mmHg}$$
$$HCO_3^- = 32 \text{ mEq/L}$$
$$BE = +2.5$$
$$SaO_2 = 78.0\%$$

Three weeks later, Mr. Spitz returns to the clinic. He says he has been feeling bad for the last 2 days with increasing cough and a mild fever. The following ABG is obtained while he is breathing 1 L/min O_2 via nasal cannula. What is your interpretation?

The PaO_2 has fallen to 49 mmHg, indicating an increasing degree of _____.

hypoxemia

The $PaCO_2$ has risen to 69 mmHg, telling us Mr. Spitz's ventilation has _____.

decreased

Gas exchange remains impaired, as evidenced by the increased _____.

A-aDO$_2$

The pH has fallen to 7.28, indicating the _____ has worsened.

acidemia

The rising $PaCO_2$ indicates a worsening of the _____ acidosis.

respiratory

The metabolic _____ is still present from his compensation for a chronically elevated $PaCO_2$.

alkalosis

This ABG confirms the diagnosis of _____ respiratory failure.

hypercapnic

Note: Acute hypercapnic respiratory failure is common in patients with underlying COPD. These patients, although disabled by their disease, are nevertheless functionally stable from day to day. The critical situation develops when some further insult such as a minor infection occurs and results in sudden worsening in gas exchange. Having no pulmonary reserve, these patients tend to develop increasing levels of hypoxemia, hypercapnia, and acidemia.

$$pH = 7.47$$

$$PaCO_2 = 38 \text{ mmHg}$$

$$PaO_2 = 94 \text{ mmHg}$$

$$HCO_3^- = 27.5 \text{ mEq/L}$$

$$BE = +4.0$$

$$SaO_2 = 97.4\%$$

Mr. Spitz's condition continued to deteriorate and he was intubated and placed on mechanical ventilation with 35 percent O_2. After 4 hours of mechanical ventilation, the above ABG was obtained. What is your interpretation?

The PaO_2 of 94 mmHg tells us that the hypoxemia has been

_____.   *corrected*

The $PaCO_2$ has been driven _____ to 38 mmHg.   *down*

Note: Do you recall what a normal ventilatory status is for Mr. Spitz? His baseline $PaCO_2$ is 50 to 55 mmHg. His disease has progressed to the point where it is normal for him to slightly hypoventilate. Bringing the $PaCO_2$ to a textbook normal level is inappropriate in this situation.

The $A\text{-}aDO_2$ remains increased, indicating _____ gas   *abnormal*
exchange.

The pH has risen to 7.47 and has become _____.   *alkaline*

Note: This ABG could be interpreted as a simple metabolic alkalosis, but we know Mr. Spitz's previous baseline ABGs. This allows us to properly interpret this current ABG as showing respiratory alkalemia due to excessive mechanical ventilation. Proper management of this patient would have been to bring ABG values to levels appropriate for his chronic and stable state of hypoventilation.

$$pH = 7.46$$
$$PaCO_2 = 56 \text{ mmHg}$$
$$PaO_2 = 58 \text{ mmHg}$$
$$HCO_3^- = 40 \text{ mEq/L}$$
$$BE = +13$$
$$SaO_2 = 90.7\%$$

Mr. Lunger is a patient with advanced COPD who is also being treated for chronic congestive heart failure. He has come into the clinic for a followup visit breathing 2 L/min O_2 via nasal cannula when the above ABG is obtained. What is your interpretation?

The PaO_2 of 58 mmHg indicates a _____ hypoxemia.   *moderate*

The $PaCO_2$ of 56 mmHg indicates the presence of alveolar
_____ .   *hypoventilation*

The A-aDO_2 is _____ , indicating the presence of a   *increased*
gas exchange abnormality.

The pH of 7.46 indicates a slight _____ .   *alkalemia*

The high $PaCO_2$ and high HCO_3^- indicates a respiratory
_____ and a metabolic _____ .   *acidosis, alkalosis*

Note: This ABG represents a mixed acid-base disturbance. Mr. Lunger has been chronically taking steroids and a diuretic for his medical problems. Both of these were promoting excess loss of K^+. This resulted in the development of a metabolic alkalosis superimposed on the metabolic compensation for his chronic respiratory acidosis. It should be obvious why interpretation of more complex acid-base disturbances requires more information than that provided with the ABG values alone. Without the knowledge of this patient's history and the medications he is taking, it would be quite difficult to properly interpret his ABGs.

$$pH = 7.49$$

$$PaCO_2 = 30 \text{ mmHg}$$

$$PaO_2 = 72 \text{ mmHg}$$

$$HCO_3^- = 22.6 \text{ mEq/L}$$

$$BE = +0.5$$

$$SaO_2 = 95.8\%$$

Ms. Brittle is a 68-year-old woman who had been hospitalized for a hip fracture. She had rather suddenly experienced shortness of breath when the above ABG results were obtained. What is your interpretation?

The PaO_2 of 72 mmHg indicates a _____ hypoxemia.   *mild*

The $PaCO_2$ of 30 mmHg indicates that she is _____.   *hyperventilating*

The A-aDO_2 is _____ mmHg, which indicates a mild gas exchange abnormality.   *40*

The pH of 7.49 indicates an _____.   *alkalemia*

The low $PaCO_2$ tells us there is a respiratory _____.   *alkalosis*

The combination of a low $PaCO_2$, high pH, and normal HCO_3^- tells us this is a _____ respiratory alkalemia.   *simple or primary*

In light of the lack of metabolic compensation, we would also refer to this as an _____ respiratory alkalosis.   *acute*

Note: This ABG pattern of acute hyperventilation with mild to moderate hypoxemia is commonly seen in patients with pulmonary emboli. Acute shortness of breath in a high-risk patient should immediately bring this possibility to mind.

Appendix B *Siggaard-Andersen Alignment Nomogram*

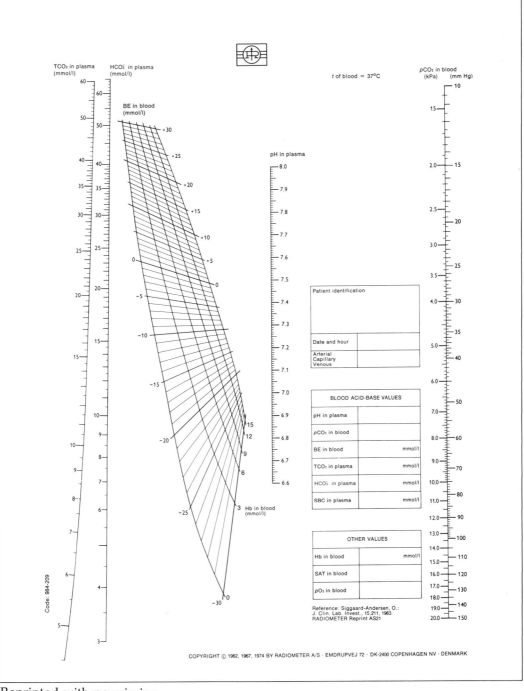

Reprinted with permission.

Glossary

Frequently Used Terms and Symbols

Term	Symbol	Definition	Normal Value
Acid		Substance that donates H^+	
Acidemia		Acidic blood	pH < 7.38
Acidosis		Condition that would tend to cause an acidemia	
Alkalemia		Alkaline blood	pH > 7.42
Alkalosis		Condition that would tend to cause an alkalemia	
Alveolar-arterial oxygen gradient	$A\text{-}aDO_2$	Alveolar-to-arterial blood oxygen difference	10–12 mmHg room air
Alveolar ventilation	V_A	Ventilation that participates in gas exchange	350 ml per breath
Anion		Negatively charged ion	
Anion gap	AG	Difference between measured cations and anions. Increased value associated with metabolic acidosis	10–16 mEq/L
Arterial blood gas	ABG	Analysis of arterial blood for pH, $PaCO_2$, PaO_2	See individual components
Arterial carbon dioxide tension	$PaCO_2$	Partial pressure of carbon dioxide in arterial blood	38–42 mmHg
Arterial oxygen content	CaO_2	Content of oxygen in arterial blood	20 cc/dl blood
Arterial oxygen saturation	SaO_2	Saturation level of arterial blood Hb with O_2	95–97%
Arterial oxygen tension	PaO_2	Partial pressure of oxygen in arterial blood	80–100 mmHg
Base		Substance that accepts H^+	
Base deficit	BD	A negative base excess value	
Base excess	BE	Difference between actual and predicted blood buffer base value	−2 to +2
Bicarbonate concentration	$[HCO_3^-]$	Bicarbonate concentration in mEq/L	22–26 mEq/L
Capnography		Analysis of exhaled gas for CO_2	
Carbon dioxide production	$\dot{V}CO_2$	Carbon dioxide produced by metabolism per minute	200 ml/min
Carbonic acid	H_2CO_3	Acid formed when CO_2 and H_2O combine	1.2 mM/L
Cation		Positively charged ion	
Compensation		The altering of function of the respiratory or renal system in an attempt to correct for an acid-base disorder	
Dead space	V_D	Ventilation that does not participate in gas exchange	1 cc/lb (anatomic)
Diffusion		Movement of a gas from area of high partial pressure to area of low partial pressure	
Diffusion defect		Impairment of gas exchange at the alveolar-capillary membrane	
Electrolyte		Ion with a positive or a negative charge	

Term	Symbol	Definition	Normal Value
Fractional inspired oxygen concentration	F_IO_2	Percent of oxygen in the air the patient is breathing	Room air = 21%
Gas exchange		Exchange of O_2 or CO_2 between lungs and blood	
Hemoglobin	Hb	Protein in red blood cell capable of carrying O_2	14–16 gm/dl
Hydrogen ion concentration	$[H^+]$	Hydrogen ion concentration in nmol/L	40 nmol/L
Hypercapnia		$PaCO_2$ above normal	$PaCO_2 > 42$ mmHg
Hyperventilation		Excessive V_A resulting in $PaCO_2$ below normal	$PaCO_2 < 38$ mmHg
Hypocapnia		$PaCO_2$ below normal	$PaCO_2 < 38$ mmHg
Hypoventilation		Decreased V_A resulting in $PaCO_2$ above normal	$PaCO_2 > 42$ mmHg
Hypoxemia		PaO_2 less than normal	$PaO_2 < 80$ mmHg
Hypoxia		Lack of adequate oxygen at the tissue level	
Minute ventilation	$\dot{V}E$	Total ventilation in 1 minute	5–10 L/min
Mixed venous carbon dioxide	$P\bar{v}CO_2$	Partial pressure of carbon dioxide in mixed venous blood	46 mmHg
Mixed venous oxygen content	$C\bar{v}O_2$	Content of oxygen in mixed venous blood (i.e., pulmonary artery)	15 cc/dl blood
Mixed venous oxygen saturation	$S\bar{v}O_2$	Saturation level of mixed venous blood Hb with O_2	75%
Mixed venous oxygen tension	$P\bar{v}O_2$	Partial pressure of oxygen in mixed venous blood	40 mmHg
Oximetry		Measurement of oxygen saturations by light-absorbance properties of oxygenated Hb	
Oxygen consumption	$\bar{V}O_2$	Oxygen consumed by metabolism per minute	250 ml/min
pH	pH	Negative log of the hydrogen ion concentration	7.38–7.42
Respiratory exchange ratio	R	Ratio of $\dot{V}CO_2/\dot{V}O_2$ measured at the lungs	0.8
Respiratory quotient	RQ	Ratio of $\dot{V}CO_2/\dot{V}O_2$ measured at the tissues	0.8
Shunt	Qs/Qt	Passage of venous blood from right side of heart to left side without exchanging gas with alveoli	3–5% of cardiac output
Tidal volume	V_T	Amount of air inspired with each breath	500 ml per breath
Transcutaneous partial pressure of carbon dioxide	$P_{tc}CO_2$	Partial pressure of carbon dioxide measured by a skin electrode	
Transcutaneous partial pressure of oxygen	$P_{tc}O_2$	Partial pressure of oxygen measured on the skin	
Ventilation		Movement of gas in and out of lungs	
Ventilation-perfusion ratio	V/Q	Ratio of alveolar ventilation to perfusion in the lungs	0.8

Index